The abuse of women within childcare work

KIERAN O'HAGAN and
KAROLA DILLENBURGER

OPEN UNIVERSITY PRESS
Buckingham · Philadelphia

Open University Press
Celtic Court
22 Ballmoor
Buckingham
MK18 1XW

and
1900 Frost Road, Suite 101
Bristol, PA 19007, USA

First Published 1995

A catalogue record of this book is available from the British Library

ISBN 0 335 19260 2 (pb)   0 335 19261 0 (hb)

Library of Congress Cataloging-in-Publication Data

Typeset by Type Study, Scarborough
Printed in Great Britain by Biddles Limited, Guildford and Kings Lynn

Contents

Part II   Manifestations

PART I

The abusive context

1

A case in point

It was precisely 2.45 p.m. when Patricia Murray opened the door of her back-to-back dingy terrace and found two strangers, a man and a woman, staring at her. Numerous possibilities came to mind: Were they selling? Canvassing for votes? Converting for God? But she sensed that none of these applied, and she suddenly felt uneasy. The woman spoke first.

'Mrs Murray, my name's Caroline Davis and this is my colleague, John Matthews; we're from the social services department; could we possibly have a word with you?'

Their smiles and friendly words did not entirely conceal a certain tension. The man in particular betrayed something ominous; the word 'social services' confirmed it.

'Social services?' Patricia asked, her mind trying to cope with anticipated trouble, and her resentment swelling as a consequence of their arrival without notice, their failed attempts to allay her fears until they got through the door. She wanted to say: 'Why didn't you let me know you were coming? . . . call back again when my husband Carl is here . . . it's not convenient . . .' etc. But she didn't. Nor could she, for two reasons: she did not have the confidence, and she sensed power and determination behind a veneer of friendliness and good intent. (Carl was her common law husband, father of her youngest child Tracy.)

'Yes that's right, Mrs Murray; we're from the North Road office. Is it okay for us to have a word? . . . it won't take long.'

'What about?' she managed to ask, yet dreading the reply. It had to be about one of her children.

The woman was about to say something, but hesitated. She had obviously not anticipated the question on the doorstep. The man unexpectedly spoke:

'We'd prefer to speak to you . . . *inside your own home*, Mrs Murray.'

This was meant to sound respectful, but Patricia's fear and anxiety increased considerably. Again, she could not say what she knew and felt: they had something grave to tell her, and they required the safety and confinement of her own living room in which to do so. They obviously felt exposed and vulnerable standing on her doorstep. Patricia now had an even greater desire to tell them to call back when she was not alone, when her children and husband would be with her; but she had even less confidence to resist them. She allowed them in.

Their tone and manner changed considerably. They checked that Carl was not there before they sat down. Then they told her. Her second oldest daughter Karen, aged 8, had alleged to her school teacher that Carl had beaten her. She had some bruising on her left arm to prove it. The schoolteacher had told the school's child abuse coordinator (a recent innovation) who had told the headteacher. Both the child abuse coordinator and the headteacher had spoken to the child and decided to inform social services. As required, social services informed the police. The police decided not to get involved at this stage. They regarded the bruise-on-the-arm referral as not very serious and agreed to social services continuing with the investigation.

Patricia listened to the social workers with a mounting sense of anger and incredulity. She tried to remember the details of the day's events as they had described them. She tried to concentrate on what was presented to her as a logical sequence of events.

They questioned her about Karen's allegation. Was she aware of it? Did she see Carl do it? Where was she when it happened? Had she ever seen him hit her before? How often and for how long was Carl left in charge of the children? Was he violent towards Patricia herself? Did he have a drink problem? What did she know of Carl's background? Was she aware that he was convicted of a charge of GBH when he was 17 (he was now 32)? What was their relationship like generally?

The questions were not asked as rapidly as this. There was a good deal of foreplay, testing out, bobbing and weaving, creating the right cue for whichever question they had in mind. They were very skilled in controlling her reactions; no matter how angry or disgusted she became, they seemed somehow able to deflate, to divert, and then to begin again. Nowhere more so than when they eventually asked Patricia to accompany them to the school, to collect Karen, to take her to the local hospital for a medical examination. She was shocked. Yet she felt impotent, because they had prefaced this request by describing the injury they had seen, testing out whether or not she was concerned and what she intended to do about it (she was very concerned and intended seeking medical attention herself). She despised their ingratiating 'we know you'll always want to do your best for your daughter, Mrs Murray'.

Patricia thought for a moment that she should knock on the wall (the traditional way of beckoning her friend and neighbour Joan when emergencies arose). But there was such potential now for trouble, for shame and stigma ('What has Carl done to her?' she herself asked angrily, and what will be the outcome?) that she decided she must go it alone for the meanwhile.

There was much haste in the departure for the school. Patricia again thought of her neighbour Joan as she descended the steps and walked towards their car. She thought of her other neighbours too; many of whom would have understood her plight and supported her, but some of whom would have been gratified. Social services were well known in this locality.

Karen was so relieved to see her mother that she burst into tears and flung her arms around her. Patricia comforted and reassured her, but she was acutely conscious of the fact that it was a spectacle for those who surrounded them. She could not rid her mind of the scene in which her child was questioned by these people when she was not there, and she wondered how honest they had been, with both her child and herself. She felt a particular empathy with Karen, recalling how she herself had felt manipulated by them in her own home; how easy it must have been for them to manipulate her child, away from home.

Karen's left upper arm was indeed bruised. In the presence of the social workers (who attempted to look as inconspicuous as possible) Karen told Patricia that it had happened last night. As was the case two nights a week, Carl was minding the three children, and Patricia was working in a downtown café. Karen and her older sister Sheila had been playing, then arguing, then fighting, and Sheila had complained. Patricia immediately recognized the pattern; she also realized that Karen, in her present state, was significantly altering some detail of the event for fear of retribution; she was a constant source of irritation to her older sister, and seemed to delight in testing out how much she could provoke her before Carl or Patricia intervened. It was all so familiar, thought Patricia, but she had never known Carl to strike her, let alone strike and leave this kind of bruising. She was appalled and angered by it, and she wanted Carl to be there that moment so that she could confront him.

She did not oppose the 'suggestion' of a medical examination but she asked could she take Karen to her own doctor. They had obviously anticipated this request, and spoke of the hospital paediatrician's expertise in dealing with this kind of injury, the possibility of fractures and 'other complications'. This was meant to reassure Patricia. But it did not. She sensed that she really had no choice in the matter, that the appointment with the paediatrician had already been made, and that it would be kept no matter what she said.

'I need to be home for my other two', she protested. But that too had been anticipated; they would collect the children with her (one of them, Catherine, attended the same school) and take them to the hospital also.

'What for?' Patricia enquired (surely not my convenience, she thought).

'It might be helpful for your other two children to be looked at too, Mrs Murray.'

For a split second, Patricia thought this was a bad dream, and that she might waken any moment. But their reasoning about their intent quickly told her otherwise: 'Abusers seldom abuse one child only, Mrs Murray . . . very often the abuse has been going on quite a while . . . children are often bribed to keep quiet.'

Patricia erupted. She yelled at them that she was not going to let her other two children be seen by anybody. Then she burst into tears, full of anger for them and remorse for her daughter, visibly shaken by her mother's outburst. They relented, though they stressed again that it was an 'excellent opportunity' for her to be reassured that whatever had happened to Karen, had not happened to her other two children.

At the hospital, Patricia and her children waited impatiently in a queue, in the midst of a noisy and crowded reception area. The receptionist asked her some questions and opened a new file. She then told Patricia to sit and listen for the child's name to be called.

The social workers sat with her. They spoke to her often, but she seldom heard them. A thousand thoughts raced through her mind. The most repetitive one was that she should not be here, and that she should simply have refused to come. They had tried to convince her that she would feel good about coming and that deep inside she knew it was the right thing to do. She did not feel good; she felt anxious, humiliated and helpless. And she was not at all convinced that it was the right thing to do. She was in no fit state either to alleviate Karen of the fear or guilt the child was feeling, nor was she able to cope with the other two children's persistent demands to know why they were there. She thought of that one explosive moment when she had asserted herself, refusing permission for them to be examined. She wondered whether or not she should have insisted that they be brought home to the care of her neighbour. It would have been convenient for both Patricia and children; but she was now determined that all her children remain with her.

The reception nurse called out her name. She resented that and got up hurriedly. She hoped the examination would be as brief as possible. But the call was a false alarm; children had to be weighed and measured before seeing the paediatrician. That took 20 minutes. Then they had to return to the reception area, and await a second call.

For whatever reason, Patricia was convinced that the paediatrician would be female. When they eventually got inside the surgery she was surprised and discomforted to find a male. Dr Marks was his name. He was warm and friendly and attempted to lessen her anxiety. He spent ten minutes or more establishing rapport with Karen. He asked Patricia many questions about her, from the time of the pregnancy, the details of the birth, Karen's subsequent development, immunizations, illnesses, diet and her present state of health generally. He looked briefly at the bruising and asked Patricia did she know anything about it. He took careful note of the way mother and daughter related to each other. He often brought Karen into the conversation and watched how Patricia responded. He could see that the relationship was a normal one, free from any underlying pervasive fear or pressure. Then he proceeded to examine her.

He began with her eyes, ears and throat. He used a lot of stimulating techniques and aids in order to do this inconspicuously and funnily. Then he asked Karen to take her top off, saying he wanted to make sure her heart 'was still beating'. He offered to let her hear it herself. He then asked her to lie on his couch. He beckoned to Patricia to stand nearby. He examined Karen's back and front from the waist upwards, and measured some faded bruising. He turned to Patricia and said he wanted to examine 'down below'; he suggested that Patricia help Karen undress. Karen stared apprehensively at her mother.

Patricia had predicted and dreaded this suggestion. From the moment she had arrived at the hospital, she had sensed that Karen would be subjected to something more than a speedy check of the bruising on her arm. The weighing and measuring and the opening of a new file had confirmed it. She appreciated the gentle and caring way he had treated Karen, the fun and games had reduced the child's distress considerably. But he seemed oblivious to the awful dilemma which his request now posed for her. She was horrified by the suggestion (implied by this next stage of the examination) that her child may also have been sexually abused. She did not want him, a man, examining her child's genitalia. She did not want any man near her child for this purpose. But she had not the confidence to say so. She would have a lot of explaining to do to Karen; she had repeatedly warned her children about the dangers of strange men generally. She had been highly effective in warning them about inappropriate touching in particular. She had made no exceptions, even for doctors.

She bit her lip and moved over to her child. 'Let's take this off', she said innocuously. But Karen looked confused and anxious, as though aware that her mother was instructing her to do something she had always told her not to do. She also sensed some contradiction between her mother's apparently innocent tone of voice and the tense pained expression on her face.

Dr Marks gently prodded Karen's stomach area. Then he asked her to open her legs wide. He put his fingers on her vulva and slightly stretched it so that he could examine a little of the vaginal canal. He moved his head very close to it. He asked Karen to turn away from him. She did not understand, and looked at her mother. With her mother's help, she turned and got herself into the foetal position. He carefully fingered and examined her anus. 'Good', he said. He looked at her thighs, knees and toes; again he measured some faded bruising. Then he looked at the bruising on her arm. It was fresh and moist. He asked her to move her arm in various directions and to tell him how it felt. He carefully measured it, took note of its varying colours, and remarked: 'I don't think too much damage has been done'.

When Karen was dressed, and they were all seated, Dr Marks told Patricia that the injuries to the arm were definitely non-accidental. The imprint of a fist could be clearly seen amidst the bruising. He confirmed that Karen's state of health generally was excellent, but he was concerned about the potential for even greater injury in the future. He asked her many questions about events around the incident, just like the social workers had done; and he attempted to explore relationships within the family generally, and between herself and Carl in particular.

Patricia was occasionally conscious of the questioning; but much more lasting in its impact was the memory of Dr Mark's fingers on her child's anus and genitalia. She was vaguely conscious of the intrusiveness of questions about her marriage and relationships; puzzled and irritated by such questions, and uncertain why. But there was nothing vague or confusing about the impact of his examination. She found it difficult to concentrate upon anything else.

The social workers brought the family home. Their friendly chat and attempts to reassure Patricia 'now that we know what the problem is, Mrs Murray', convinced her they were light years away from her state of mind and her aching head. They told her about 'procedures': the police would be informed; Carl would have to be seen; a 'case conference'(?) would be held; they would be invited to attend, etc. They asked her how Carl might react? Did she think he would pick on Karen even more? They asked her how did she feel about Carl hitting Karen? Did she find it hard to believe? Was she annoyed or angered?

Patricia could barely respond. She wished only that she could be alone for a short while. But they continued questioning her, and when the man asked her did she think Karen would 'be safe in the home tonight', she suddenly realized what they were hinting at, and exploded:

'For Christ sake ... have you not done enough ... have I not suffered enough ... I wasn't even there when it happened! You're not taking her ... you're not ... YOU'RE NOT!'

For the second time that day, Karen ran to her mother. They clasped each other tightly and wept. The social workers left soon after. They told her Carl would have to be interviewed by police and social workers.

Within the next few days, Carl was interviewed and denied the charge. Patricia supported him, despite the medical report from Dr Marks. Police and social workers attempted to speak to Karen, but the child appeared to have forgotten the incident completely. Patricia removed Karen from her school and enrolled her in another, a good deal further away.

Karen's maternal grandmother phoned social services and complained bitterly about her grandchild being made to undress by a male stranger (highly respected paediatrician though he was). She said that 'the lot of yous' (that is, social workers, police and paediatrician) had made fools of the whole family; she and family members had repeatedly warned Karen about strange men touching her in private parts. Now Karen was telling all her friends in the street and at the school about this strange man 'sticking his finger up there'.

Neither parent attended the case conference. It was decided to register Karen's name on the child abuse register. The problem of contact and monitoring was left to the discretion of the team leader and social worker.

2

The problem has not gone away

Introduction

The history of childcare work is also a history of the abuse of women perpetrated by childcare agencies. The 'abuse of women' is perhaps an idea running against the current tide. Some may think women are doing nicely, thank you. So much so that men are fighting back and alarming feminists who warn of the backlash (Faludi 1992; French 1993; Figes 1994). Whatever the present state of play, the indisputable fact is that during the last three decades women have been hurt, humiliated, deceived, frightened, undermined, let down, coerced, endangered, impoverished, and stigmatized, by childcare professionals working for childcare and child protection agencies. More importantly, the causes of that abuse remain, and the abuses are still occurring. This text will argue that certain categories of abuses are actually increasing in their occurrence. Many professionals are unaware of the abuse they perpetrate against women; it is seldom intentional abuse. Some are aware, but are motivated by a greater preoccupation with the welfare of the child. Childcare workers often perceive a conflict of interest between the rights of a mother and the welfare of her child. They may question the validity of a book devoted primarily to how childcare agencies treat women; they may believe that the only essential question is how such agencies treat children. But the authors share a conviction that to abuse the mother (or any other primary carer) of a child is to abuse the child also, and that the quality of care provided for the child is greatly affected by how professionals think about, approach, and respond to the child's principal carer. This conviction is based upon abundant evidence in research, childcare literature, and in our combined experiences of nearly forty years of frontline childcare work. The perceived conflict between the welfare of the child and the rights of a mother is central in any discussion about the abuse of women; it will be referred to and explored throughout this text. The abuse of women takes many forms. Later chapters will explore common and easily perpetrated abuses. This chapter will explore the belief shared by many that effective safeguards now exist, ensuring that such abuses are a thing of the past.

Safeguards

The suggestion that childcare workers frequently abuse women in the course of their work provokes controversy and resentment, for sound reasons. First, childcare workers are dedicated, committed people, who enter childcare with the best possible motives. They achieve success on a daily basis, and thousands of families and children are grateful to them. Second, the vast majority of frontline childcare workers – that is, social workers, health visitors, midwives, police officers (assigned to child abuse teams), etc. – are women (Norris, 1991). They do not consciously and willingly abuse women, and they are better equipped in empathy, experience, and awareness, enabling them to avoid abusing women. Dobrin's (1989) research suggests that professional women in childcare make decisions which are more ethically sound than those made by their male colleagues. Third, past abuses of women clients in childcare work are no secret; all professionals are aware of it and of the present-day vulnerability of women facing child abuse investigations alone. There are also many child abuse enquiry reports which have identified how the mothers of alleged and actual victims of abuse have been systematically abused as a consequence of professional negligence, incompetence and deception (DHSS 1974; Greenwich 1987; Butler-Sloss 1988). Surely then, the consequence of all this awareness of the abuse of women is to increase vigilence which prevents it?

Fourth, the various professions involved in childcare have evolved ethical codes, the sole purpose of which is to ensure that professionals *do not abuse any client in any way.* Fifth, new laws and government guidelines, in particular the Children Act 1989, emphasize parental duties and re-sponsibilities, and the duty on the part of childcare agencies, of upholding them. Sixth, childcare agencies responsible for child protection work pro-vide comprehensive procedures derived from these new laws and guide-lines. The procedures are usually prefaced by principles derived from the agencies' ethical codes and anti-discriminatory policies. All childcare agen-cies now have official complaints procedures too, enabling any client to expose whatever abuse may have been perpetrated against them. Seventh, feminist literature has widespread readership and approval among child-care workers, the vast majority of whom are women; feminists have been very influential in exposing the oppression of women in general, and the sexual abuse of women and children in particular. One may reasonably conclude therefore, that feminism would be an effective bulwark against any form of abuse of women in childcare work. Eighth, training for child protection work has improved dramatically. Courses today contain components which aim to equip professionals for confronting discrimination in all its forms. Many trainers are preoccupied with gender discrimination. The training also facilitates self-exploration which can help future professionals identify events and experiences in their past and characteristics of their own personalities, either or both of which may be conducive to them unwittingly abusing women. Finally, women who believe they have been abused as parents by childcare agencies have found their own solution in uniting, sharing their experiences, advertising their existence, and successfully forming pressure groups which monitor as best they can, current practices in childcare work.

Limitations of 'safeguards'

Let us look more closely at these safeguards and at some factors which may impinge upon them.

Integrity of childcare workers

Childcare is a profession demanding discipline, commitment, integrity, patience, tolerance, courage and a sense of humour. Anyone involved in childcare, in training, practice, or management, is perfectly justified in believing in the essential goodness of childcare workers. Does this goodness not therefore constitute the most effective safeguard against them doing harm by abusing women? Unfortunately, no. Childcare workers daily encounter powerful and influential forces which make it difficult and sometimes impossible to adhere to their own high moral standards, and to the non-discriminatory principles and practice they may have adopted through training and experience. These forces exist in childcare agencies, in the communities those agencies serve, and, in the wider local and national political context. Abusive actions, however, do not always originate in these wider contexts; the sheer complexity and danger of many childcare cases often leads to action and decision making which are abusive in their effects. Finally, as in any profession, some childcare workers are seriously flawed and lack many of the qualities mentioned above. They are well capable of abusing any group of clients.

Gender

The vast majority of frontline childcare workers are women, but the majority of those who manage and supervise them are men (Hearn 1990;

Grimwood and Popplestone 1993). This gender factor may or may not be significant in determining the extent of abuse perpetrated against mothers. Howe *et al.* (1988) believe that gender and personal history impinges upon judgements made in childcare work. It may be that women are more strongly motivated by the abuse of a child than they are concerned about the potential abuse of a mother. Some feminist writers (Sayers 1991; Lawrence 1992) suggest that processes of memory, emotion, and counter-transference may cause women in childcare to abuse women clients. This is a serious charge, and will be explored in more depth in Chapter 5.

The perspective and response of many of the new, career-led managers (overwhelmingly male) who have occupied key positions in health and social services during the past decade is markedly different from that of their frontline staff (Kirwan 1994). They are seldom as empathic or as sensitive to mothers; nor are they as likely to be aware of the numerous ways in which the actions they dictate can be abusive. The pressures which bear down upon managers can widen or constrict their focus of concern. It is widened if it goes beyond consideration of the welfare of the child and the rights of the mother (to consider for example, issues like financial costs, availability of resources, statistical returns, etc.). It can be constricted by a preoccupation, even an obsession, with the question of whether or not the child is being abused. One of the primary goals of childcare managers is the minimization of risk; but not just risk to the child, they are equally concerned about risk to their own and their department's reputation. Every experienced frontline child protection worker can recall supervisory sessions in which their managers have revealed this concern to an unhelpful extent. BBC2's (1992) controversial play *Bad Girl* is a case in point: the social work team leader is grilled by his manager and reminded of the death of a child; he is also sent unmistakable messages about the consequences if another case goes the same way. The team leader gets very anxious about another case; his anxiety underpins the pressure he applies to the increasingly disillusioned female social worker, and the shocking abuses of the single parent mother which follow. Such anxiety is often a strait-jacket from which some managers never escape, particularly if they have had a 'close shave' with a child abuse fatality in the past. The female social worker in that play resigned. She realized that the 'service' she was offering the mother was no service at all. Many childcare workers know precisely how she felt and would agree with Statham (1987) and Hudson *et al.* (1994) who emphasize that the ferocity of cutbacks in welfare provision as a whole, compel women professionals at the frontline to deliver to women clients a service they know to be wholly inadequate at best, and abusive in the long term.

Awareness

Awareness of the abuses of women, and of how professionals have actually abused women in the past, should minimize such abuses in the present and future. The problem is that awareness seldom lasts, and that its influence diminishes quickly in the stress laden, dilemma-riddled problems that are the lot of frontline childcare workers. To be faced with the question of whether or not an infant has been subjected to whiplash shaking, or whether or not a five year old has been buggered, or, whether or not a disabled teenager is being emotionally abused (and, if so, what precisely is going to be done about it; what emergency legislation to invoke; which alternative accommodation to find; what care proceedings to pursue?) – such immediate problems and the inevitable risks inherent in each proposed solution can easily eradicate any memory or awareness of abuses perpetrated by professionals against the carers of such children. As the emphasis understandably fixes on the child and risk to the child, so shifts the focus from the parent/carer, their domestic/marital context, economic and social factors etc., all of which should remain important areas to explore in assessment. Worse than ignoring them, however, is when certain features of any of them actually become the instrument of abuse. For example, 'single parenthood' may from the outset, be perceived negatively; rather than exploring the difficulties encountered by a single parent mother, and how the agencies may alleviate her of any hardships conducive to the dynamics and attitudes leading to child abuse (as they are statutorily obliged to do, s. 17, Children Act, 1989), some professionals may merely want to concentrate on the adverse impact of the hardships upon the mother's caring abilities: 'she can't provide proper care for those kids ... she's never in ... she works six nights a week ... she's too tired to manage ... she's no support in the street ... never gets on with folk ... but she'll let any old Tom, Dick or Harry look after the kids'. These are all common prejudices which may be consciously expressed by professionals fully aware of the potential abuse of the mother which they may constitute, yet much more aware and affected by their belief that the risk to the child is unacceptably high.

Awareness may do nothing to prevent the abuse of women if the professional is driven by an ideological fervour which in itself is demonstrably abusive. Such ideology and its disastrous impact has been much in evidence in childcare in recent years (Statham 1987; King and Trowell 1992). Some professionals may be motivated and guided by ideological and personal convictions, which, rather than alerting them to the constant possibility of their abusing women and thus preventing them from doing so, actually ensures that they will abuse women, deliberately and consciously.

Finally, awareness of the abuse of women may be gained from reading some of the 40 child abuse enquiry reports which have been produced during the past two decades. But who remembers them? Who wants to remember them? We have encountered many professionals in our own career who intentionally avoid these reports, or condemn them even without reading them. Senior practitioners were castigated in the Rochdale enquiry (Justice Brown 1991) for not having read the Cleveland report (Butler-Sloss 1988). The cost of these enquiries is understandably a source of much irritation; to read of some QC's fees of £250,000 per enquiry when childcare workers may struggle for a £20 handout is not likely to make any report a source of inspiration to workers. But, as we shall discover later, some of them provide excellent learning material on the abuse of women by childcare professionals. Professionals still abuse women today in precisely the same manner as they did in the events leading up to the death of Maria Colwell, more than 20 years ago. Little wonder though, as the dust gathers on that and many of the subsequent, equally informative but unread reports.

Ethical codes

All professional codes of ethics pledge opposition to any kind of abuse of clients or of any member of their families (for example, BMA 1983; BASW 1988; UKCC 1992). Yet the principles which such codes enunciate are often so general and platitudinous that they offer little in terms of (1) understanding the problem to which they may be applied and (2) guiding childcare workers through the ethical minefields which many childcare dilemmas constitute. One could be excused for reading the codes and not realizing any such minefields exist; nor realizing the delicate balance the childcare worker has to maintain between differing and sometimes conflicting interests; nor indeed, realizing the risks and dangers inherent in any decisions they make. Social work codes may emphasize the welfare of the child as paramount, but they say not a whit about the extent to which the rights of the parent may be sacrificed in maintaining the paramountcy of that welfare principle. Indeed, there have been many references to 'our professional code of ethics' and to this paramountcy principle (now enshrined in the Children Act), to justify actions blatantly abusive of women in recent, well publicized cases. Gillon (1992) sees fundamental shortcomings in all professional codes of ethics: they are seldom as morally self-sufficient as some may claim them to be; they often derive from laws and societal attitudes which are forever transient. There is no reason, therefore, to believe that the codes of ethics of childcare professionals will prevent women from being abused.

The Children Act

The Children Act has been referred to as an 'abusing parent's charter'. The reason for this is that many of its stipulations have been interpreted as obstacles placed in the way of protecting children from abusive parents (a serious misinterpretation of the Act). Since the Act came into force, childcare agencies, particularly social services, have had to tread very carefully if they wish to make a case about 'inadequate parenting'; they have to be much more thorough in their assessments before applying to the courts for protective and/or care orders. They have to assess not just the issue of safety, but also the welfare of the child as a whole. Most crucially of all, if they request removal of the child, they must convince the court that the alternative accommodation and quality of care they are going to provide is superior to that provided by the parents, particularly the mother. Does all this therefore not constitute an important safeguard preventing the abuse of parents generally and mothers in particular? The frank answer is that it did not prevent the abuses which were described in Chapter 1. The fact is that the Children Act gives local authorities even more discretion for potentially abusive actions by childcare workers. That potential will be explored in Chapters 6 and 11 within the context of abusive childcare systems.

Procedures

Child protection necessitates the establishment of Area Child Protection Committees, consisting of representatives from all childcare and child protective agencies. These committees have produced child protection procedural handbooks to which they expect their staff to adhere. Management will contend that there is a strong moral and legal underpinning to these procedures, ensuring that ethical codes and laws are upheld, and that all those with whom the staff from the differing agencies come into contact, will be treated in accordance with anti-discriminatory policy generally. The problem is, that different Area Child Protection Committees in different parts of the UK have interpreted childcare laws and principles in different ways, thus leading to much diversity in the way their procedural handbooks are written, and consequently, how the procedures are put into effect in practice. The principle of 'partnership with parents' for example, is being applied with vigour and conviction in some areas, and being perceived as a threat in others. Parents are permitted to attend whole case conferences and/or, they are permitted to attend only for the briefest period, that is, a few minutes at the beginning, then five or ten minutes to hear the results at the end. Parents may be informed promptly and comprehensively of allegations made against them, or, they may be kept entirely in the dark even if professional childcare workers have made the allegations and wish to remain anonymous. Single parent mothers are much more vulnerable to this diversity; they are the primary carers and often the only carer to face the professionals. The procedural handbooks which some professionals are compelled to adhere to, rather than ensuring fair play to women, can actually be an instrument of abuse against them.

All local authority social services departments have official complaints procedures, enabling any member of the public to register dissatisfaction with the service offered. But as any staff member will acknowledge, such procedures are enormously complicated, time consuming, protracted, and demanding the maximum degree of assertiveness and determination on the part of those courageous enough to complain. The Family Rights Group (FRG) certainly has not been impressed by complaints procedures (Rickford 1992; Jackson 1993). The average inarticulate, unconfident, poverty-stricken, single parent mother is not likely to be able to take advantage of them. Furthermore, local authorities do not make too much effort to advertise these potentially critical facilities. O'Hagan (1994b) found that parents were totally unaware of a new policy on parental participation which had been in operation for one year.

Feminism and feminist literature

The feminist movement and feminist literature has been central to the growing awareness of the structural oppression and abuse of women. More specifically, they have 'challenged the perception that their abuse of children is their personal problem, rather than linked to the conditions in which they live' (Parton 1990: 47). Feminism has been a principal driving force in the exposure of child sexual abuse. This exposure depended primarily not upon feminist dogma and ideology, but on the testimonies of sexually abused women for whom feminists more than anyone else, provided refuge, support and counselling. This is an important point to make: actual face-to-face contact with women victims, listening to and caring for them, recording their case histories and the consequences of the sexual and other abuses they endured – these experiences are what gave credibility to feminist claims about the prevalency of child sexual abuse. It imbued feminists with a near missionery zeal to expose it and a conviction that sexual abuse was the worst possible kind of abuse (O'Hagan 1989). We have worked with many colleagues professing allegience to feminist principles and ideals, and exercising them in a way for which abused children are justifiably grateful. But we have also encountered feminists who share the view that some women are responsible for the abuse perpetrated by their partners, because they know that their partners are persistently violent or perversely sexual, and yet remain with them; almost inevitably, the child(ren) will be violently and perversely abused too. Such convictions lead to 'child-centred' policy and practice (Richardson and Bacon 1991). Those who adopt this policy believe that children must be 'rescued' and 'protected' from such abuse at all costs, even though, ironically, women, as mothers, would often be the principal victims of a vigorous rescue and protection policy, and their children would likely suffer serious emotional and psychological damage in the process (O'Hagan 1993). The stark reality is that even if 'protection by removal' was a sensible, viable policy for abused children, local authorities remain bereft of a reasonable quality of alternative accommodation and care which has to be provided.

Feminist literature displays little awareness of, or interest in, the women-abusive minutiae of childcare work. It has not for example, provided women with strategies enabling them to identify and to resist the subtle and not-so-subtle methods used in child abuse investigations (as demonstrated in Chapter 1). Feminist influence has also been conspicuously lacking in exposing the many abuses of women in adoption work. Howe *et al.* (1992) suggest a reason for this:

> Birth mothers have not become a cause among feminists. Birth mothers have not appeared in the pages of those who write so strongly and eloquently about women's lives. It is as if birth mothers' dilemmas confuse those who wish to think clearly and consistently about women and the relationship to children and motherhood. (p. 104)

The feminist perspective is painted with a very broad brush; its proponents wish to concentrate upon the structural, political, theoretical and historical underpinnings of the oppression of women (for example, McLeod and Dominelli 1982; Dominelli and McLeod 1989; Langan 1991a; Hudson *et al.* 1994). Such concentration is soundly based and this text has been positively influenced by it. But there are countless abuses perpetrated against women which are unlikely to be exposed through maintaining that broadest of perpectives.

Training

Training for childcare work has improved in the last decade. The content of training relevant to the abuse of women, however, is too theoretical and generalized to enlighten workers about the precise nature of such abuse. 'Gender' and 'gender oppression' are liberally taught in some courses, though under the all-embracing concept of anti-discriminatory practice. The structural and institutional oppression of women is sometimes tackled, and sexist thought, language and actions in society generally are repeatedly exposed. The teaching may be aided by numerous innovatory exercises, such as role reversal (that is, women role playing men and men role playing women, making decisions affecting the lives of women). These are important lessons, but they seldom impinge upon the specific context of the abuse of women by childcare agencies; indeed, there is little awareness in training courses of the precise means by which childcare workers consciously and unconsciously abuse women, and even less on how such abuse can be prevented (the title of this book has often had to be repeated and explained to listeners, as though it sounds so bizarre that it must be unreal, or mean something else; a sound indicator of the inadequacy of training).

Social work is at the centre of childcare work. Social work training is now a joint responsibility (referred to as 'partnership') between agencies (for example, social services, voluntary organizations, etc.) and training establishments. The agencies influence every aspect of training; they actually participate in the assessment of academic as well as practice standards. This transfer of power and responsibility has not been reciprocated; training establishments have little or no influence upon agencies, upon either their policies or their practice. Training establishments do, of course, produce the qualified people who will staff and eventually manage social services, and they are likely to leave college imbued with a strong ethical code which will inhibit them from abusing clients in any way. But much can happen in the move from academia to an agency with statutory childcare responsibilities. Childcare agencies have for decades unwittingly abused mothers supposedly in the interests of protecting children. The fact that such agencies have acquired considerable influence in the training of social workers and will be their principal employers, does not suggest that such abuses will quickly cease. Carter *et al.* (1992) lament 'the potential drift towards increasing agency management control of social work education' and remark 'it is not encouraging for anti-discriminatory education and practice' (p. 114).

Pressure groups

Costly and damaging interventions by childcare agencies have contributed to the establishment of parental pressure groups whose principal aims are to support parents, particularly mothers who have suffered as a consequence of such interventions, and to monitor current childcare work. Examples of such groups are The Family Rights Group, Parents Against Injustice (PAIN), and Parents' Aid. The National Council for One Parent Families is a much larger, longer established, more powerful pressure group; its aims are broader, but it maintains a keen interest in childcare policy and practice generally. All these groups are run in the main by women, many of whom have suffered from insensitivity or over-reaction by professionals. They have, on occasions, attempted to influence childcare legislation and policy. PAIN has gained much experience and developed expertise in the narrower child protection field; it has commissioned research into the initial and long-term effects of inappropriate investigations and interventions by agencies (Westminster College 1992); and has been present and made representations during the hearings of many recent public enquiries.

These pressure groups are an enormous source of support for women. They provide detailed accounts of the suffering many women have endured when involved with childcare agencies. They help to monitor the application of existing childcare laws and policies, and they can quickly pinpoint professional deviation from set procedures leading to the abuse of women. However, pressure groups do not prevent such abuse happening. Events in Rochdale (Justice Brown 1991) indicate so, coming as they did shortly after the report by Butler-Sloss (1988) on the Cleveland affair, in which precisely the same incompetence and ultimate abuse of mothers (and families as a whole) took place. Had anyone involved in the Rochdale scandal paid the slightest attention to PAIN's contribution to the Cleveland enquiry, it is highly unlikely that the events in Rochdale would have occurred. PAIN made its views known at both enquiries (1987, 1990a), but was in effect merely repeating itself.

Pressure groups are neither liked nor trusted by many childcare professionals. We can recall the contempt in which some pressure groups (PAIN in particular) were held by some colleagues. They are often perceived as bodies hell-bent on making life difficult for professionals, run by people obsessed by a sense of injustice stemming from some irrelevant and ancient abuse in the past. Entrenchment and obstacles are created by such perceptions. Pressure groups are kept at a distance. Group members seldom have an opportunity to explore the causes of the abuses they may have suffered. Professionals deny they abuse anyone, deny even their capability to abuse anyone, thus agencies and pressure groups remain polarized, and the abuses of women continue.

Conclusion

All nine 'safeguards' mentioned at the outset have limitations in the degree to which they can protect women from childcare agencies. The fact that the majority of childcare workers are women is no guarantee that they will not abuse women clients. The reason why and the way women professionals may abuse women clients will be explored in Chapter 5. Increasing publicity and awareness about the abuse of women in earlier public enquiries has not prevented similar abuses in later enquiries. Ethical codes are often too general and platitudinous to pinpoint the many different ways that women may be abused; clearly, the abuse of women is unethical, but many abusive actions may escape the moral censor of ethical codes steeped in a language of ambiguity and a syrupy 'fairness to one and all'. The Children Act has not turned out to be the 'Abusing Parents' Charter that some predicted; on the contrary, some features of the Act have the potential to sustain and add to the existing abuses perpetrated against women. Procedural handbooks provided by management to frontline staff often derive from childcare law and ethical codes; but those who formulate them have the same tendency to generalize and platitudinize; the handbooks provide far too much scope for (mis)interpretation; therein, as we will see, lies much potential for abusing women. Feminism and feminist literature has been instrumental in the fight against violence and sexual abuse perpetrated against women. Childcare has been more problematic for some feminists, who see a stark dichotomy between the welfare of the child and the rights of the mother. Some feminist writers advocate vigorous policies of 'rescue' and 'protection' of children, despite the evidence that both children and mothers suffer enormously. The training of childcare workers is increasingly under the influence of the very same childcare and child protective agencies which have been responsible for so much abuse of women in the past. Pressure groups have provided much support for abused women, but they have not had sufficient understanding of, nor access to, the principal sources and causes of such abuse.

The way forward

In this book, we aim to explore, understand and challenge the abuse of women. Understanding necessitates approaching the subject from various perpectives. In Chapter 3 we argue that one of the reasons why childcare workers target women for their intervention can be found in the traditional role expectation of women. We will focus on the relationship between women and their partners, their children, and other adults. Traditional role expectations are outlined and changes which have occurred in women's roles are explored. In Chapter 4 we argue that another reason underlying the abuse of women is the inadequacy of some of the dominant theories underpinning childcare work; we contend that they are outdated and potentially abusive to women when they are rigidly applied in childcare practice. Chapters 5 and 6 concentrate upon an idea commonly referred to as the 'abusive childcare system'. Is there such a thing? These two chapters explore possible origins of this idea and develop the argument that not only is it a tenable concept but also that it is a living reality, incorporating multiple layers of potentially abusive factors such as common beliefs, prevailing public and political climates, and specific childcare laws, policies, procedures and practices. Chapter 7 explores the abuse of women generally, equating much of that abuse with an abuse of power. Sexual harassment, domestic violence and rape are common examples of that abuse of power. Each of those categories of abuse will be addressed.

The abuse of women occurs throughout all phases of childcare work; Chapter 8 will provide many examples of such abuse, using actual case histories. The diverse origins of the abuses will also be explained and illustrated. One of the most common practices in childcare work is the avoidance of men. Chapter 9 will demonstrate that the consequences of this avoidance often constitutes a serious and dangerous abuse of women; it can be equally abusive and dangerous to the child, as many of the child abuse enquiry reports indicate. In Chapter 10, a new approach to childcare theory will be mapped out. Modern childcare theory can no longer exclude men from childcare work. A non-abusive, anti-discriminatory theory, based on scientific research data, will be provided. It will offer methods and techniques aimed at improving the situation for children, parents and the childcare workers who seek to serve them. Chapter 11 will suggest changes in many of the components of abusive childcare systems. These changes would greatly minimize the potential for abusing women within these systems. The final chapter will consider the implications for trainers of childcare professionals.

3

Women in society: changing roles and responsibilities

Introduction

Throughout history women have been disadvantaged, disregarded, abused and discriminated against, not only by childcare agencies but within society as a whole. The exact manifestations of discrimination differ culturally. In Western cultures women were discriminated against by being fitted to specific roles (Seward and Williamson 1970). Women had to adhere to role expectations that were clearly prescribed, limited and offered little room for change. They were to bear and rear children, look after husbands and care for the sick. They were to be good mothers, wives and carers. Female children were taught throughout their childhood that they were to fulfil these roles when they grew up. Seldom, if ever, have women been viewed in their own right, have their opinions been sought or their skills been valued in any other area.

In this chapter we will argue that one of the main reasons why women, rather than men, are targeted by childcare workers lies in this role expectation, in the historical role of women as main carers for children. Childcare workers, the majority of whom are women, have this historical role expectation in common with women clients. The fact that they have chosen childcare work for their career proves the point. Childcare workers seem to have taken the typically female role on board. However, the discussion in the previous chapter has shown that this does not prevent abuse of women clients.

We will explore aspects of the role of women in society that are relevant to the abuse of women in childcare work. Common themes emerge for workers as well as clients: women's relationship with men and their roles as wives and partners; women's relationship with children and their roles as mothers; women's relationship with other adults and their roles in employment and leisure. We will map out some of the most pertinent changes that have occurred in recent history and analyse how much of these changes have filtered through into the daily life of women clients and childcare workers.

Roles and relationships

The phrase 'the role of women in society' is usually greeted with knowing nods. Yes, I know what you mean. The Germans put it in a nutshell. They characterize the role of women with three Ks: *Kinder* (children), *Küche* (kitchen), *Kirche* (church). But is it really that simple? Is it really that easy to define women's role? Do we even know what it means to have a role? Are roles static or do they change? Can someone have more than one role? Are there any common features between roles? Questions like these need to be addressed before we can look at specific aspects of women's role in society.

The answer to the first question ('Is it really that simple?') is: no. This chapter is devoted to an analysis of the changing roles of women and the effect of these changes on childcare work. The complexity of this will become apparent as the chapter unfolds. For now it is sufficient to say that it is not that simple. Roles are much more complex. The next question, about the meaning of roles, leads us straight into the maze. It identifies the need for a definition. The dictionary offers a good starting point. 'Role' is defined as 'the part played by a person in a particular social setting' (*Collins English Dictionary* 1991). This definition incorporates two main aspects of what it means to have a role: 'playing a part' means doing something, behaving in a certain way; 'in a particular social setting' means that there are other people involved, certain other people. 'Playing a part in a particular social setting', therefore, means behaving in a certain way in relation to certain other people, in relationships with certain other people.

This definition of role is essentially the same as the definition of relationship. People are said to have relationships when they behave in certain ways with each other (*Collins English Dictionary* 1991). The behaviour in a relationship is usually a little more flexible than the behaviour expected when someone is fulfilling a role. Role behaviour is often clearly prescribed and tightly controlled. For example, the behaviour expected of someone who is playing the role of childcare worker is clearly defined by statutory obligations and codes of conduct; it is controlled by a hierarchical structure of accountability. The behaviour expected in a casual friendship is usually more flexible. However, the fact is that both terms, role and relationship, are used to describe certain patterns of behaviour between certain people.

Effects of behaviour

When people play roles and/or have relationships, the behaviour of both people is important. Neither one can be viewed in a vacuum. The interaction between both people is crucial. The behaviour of each person has an effect on the behaviour of the other. Each person is changed by the other person's behaviour. The changes may be obvious and observable. For example, someone laughs when a person tells a joke, or someone sits down when a person offers a chair. They may be hardly noticeable and not observable from the outside. For example, someone feels sad when a person breaks bad news, or someone has a thought sparked off by something a person said. Essentially, however, one person is affected, changed by the other person's behaviour. Behaviour in this context does not only mean obvious, observable behaviour. Feeling and thinking are also behaviours which are affected, changed. Relationships or roles are characterized by the fact that feelings and thinking, as well as other more obvious behaviours, of one person are influenced by the behaviour of another person.

The relationship and role of childcare workers and clients are no different. The behaviour of the childcare worker changes and influences the behaviour of the client and vice versa. But are childcare workers always aware of the changes that their behaviour produces? Are they always in control of these changes? Do they always intend them? How do childcare workers conduct the relationship with their clients? How do they fulfil their roles? How do clients respond? How do they feel? Childcare workers are not expected to be able to answer these questions or to conduct relationships with clients without training. In fact, they spend much time in their basic and post-qualifying training on learning how to create good relationships with clients.

Learning to relate

The fact that relationship building is an important factor in the syllabus of childcare training is based on the observation that relating to others is learnt behaviour. Learning how to behave in relationships starts early in life (see discussion of social development in the next chapter) and continues as long as we live. Each time we meet a new person we learn how to behave in relation to this particular person using skills acquired in past experiences, in past relationships. The same is obviously true for the other person. Relationships are accumulations of both people's previous experiences. Their behaviour is influenced by a wide range of factors such as class, race, age, disability, as well as sexual orientation. Consequently, we behave differently in each relationship, we have different relationships with different people.

Behaviour in relationships, however, does not only depend on past learning, but it also depends on the present situation. For example, if childcare worker and client meet for the first time in a crisis situation their behaviour will be different from that if they meet in a less critical situation. Both worker and client behaviour depends on past experiences and the present situation. Furthermore, their behaviour, their relationship, their role is not static. It changes. Depending on the circumstances in which childcare workers find themselves, their interaction with clients is affected. A playschool referral can turn into a child abuse investigation, a housing application can turn into a child being taken into care. Depending on the situation, the role of the worker changes. The expectations on their conduct as well as their behaviour in relation to the client is influenced. Client behaviour is affected by these changes and worker behaviour is affected by client response. It is an interactive process.

Focus on women

Most of the arguments and examples so far are true for men as well as women. Both men and women play roles in relation to other people. Both have to learn the behaviour necessary for their roles (Belotti 1975). Both are affected by the behaviour of others. Both develop different patterns of behaviour with different people and for both these patterns can change. For both, role expectations are culturally defined (Whitelegg *et al.* 1982; Lorber and Farrell 1991; Charles 1993).

One of the main reasons why childcare workers focus intervention or investigation on women is that the task of childcare is enshrined in the role of women. Expectations of women's behaviour in regard to their children are clearly defined (Miller 1976; Hanmer and Statham 1988). Women are to be the main carers for children, especially very young children. Consequently, when there are concerns about the care or control of children, mothers, rather than fathers, are held accountable. French (1993) identified the cultural context of these expectations: 'In a patriarchy, women must be mothers and they, not men, are held responsible for failures in parenting' (p. 151).

To understand the position of women in childcare work means to look at the roles and relationships of women in more detail. Childcare workers are not the only people with whom women clients have relationships. Women who become clients of childcare workers have relationships with their partners, their children, their parents or carers, their friends, their neighbours and many other people. They behave differently in each of these relationships and are changed by them in different ways. At the same time, clients are not the only people to whom childcare workers relate. Childcare workers, too, have many relationships apart from those they establish with clients (Walton 1975). Childcare workers, also, are affected by these relationships.

Relationships with adult partners

For most people the relationship they have with their adult partner is influential and important. Traditionally, in Western societies, this relationship was heavily regulated and institutionalized. Women and men were to get married. Marriages were to be monogamous. Any other kind of intimate relationship, such as homosexuality, cohabitation, or polygamous marriage, was either legally or morally prohibited. Choice of partner as well as behaviour within the partnership were clearly defined. Women were expected to marry men who were older, taller and somewhat better qualified and wealthier than themselves (McGoldrick 1989). Women were to care and nourish; men were to provide and protect. Marriage was supposed to be the ultimate goal for every woman.

Recent research has shown that traditional marriage arrangements are not working as effectively as is often portrayed. One in every three marriages ends in divorce (Hanmer and Statham 1988). Unfaithfulness and adultery is increasing for both husbands and wives (Dennis 1993). Serial monogamy (marriage–divorce–remarriage) is growing – 80 per cent of people under 30 years of age remarry soon after divorce (Hanmer and Statham 1988). The number of women who decide to marry later is increasing. Only 25 per cent of women marry before the age of 20 (McGoldrick 1989). Twenty-six per cent of couples live together before getting married (Hanmer and Statham 1988). The number of women who decide not to marry at all is growing – 12 per cent compared with 3 per cent of their parents' generation (McGoldrick 1989). Lesbian couples are becoming increasingly visible (Hanmer and Statham 1988).

Commonalties and differences between clients and workers

These trends have left neither clients nor childcare workers untouched. Many of the experiences are common to clients and workers (Hanmer and Statham 1988). Women workers and women clients experience divorce, widowhood, cohabitation, remarriage, and homosexual relationships. Some decide to marry late in life, others not to marry at all. The main difference between workers and clients is that the client's relationship with adult partners becomes open to investigation. For example, women clients are criticized if they do not live with the natural father of their children. They are criticized if they change partners frequently. They are challenged if they have lesbian relationships. They are held responsible if their partner abuses their children. Adult partnerships of workers are not open for investigation. They are private. The only times they are discussed with clients are when the worker decides that this kind of self-disclosure is appropriate.

The investigation of adult relationships of women clients is usually based on the evidence of the women. Women are asked how they are getting on with their husband/boyfriend. Does he like the kids? Is he violent (see Chapter 6)? Does he help in the house? Is he moving in/out? Childcare workers tend to avoid asking the adult partner himself (see Chapter 8). As Hanmer and Statham (1988) put it 'men figure prominently in the lives of many women clients and may even be identified as a major problem for the women clients, but social work intervention is either seen as inappropriate or impossible' (p. 68).

Relationships with children

Another common experience for women clients as well as women workers is having children. Eighty per cent of all women have children (Hanmer and Statham 1988). The percentage of men who have children may be similar; however, exact figures are much more difficult to obtain. Traditionally, maternal rather than paternal care was viewed the key to bringing up children (Hanmer and Statham 1988). Expectations of women's behaviour were clearly defined, especially while the children were very young. First and foremost, women were to be homemakers and carers. McGoldrick (1989) found that 'the expectation for women has been that they would take care of the needs of others, first men, then children, then the elderly' (p. 29).

Women were to conform to these expectations within the context of the family. Oakley (1982) describes: ' "The family" in its attenuated, conventionalised form (two parents, 2.4 children, father breadwinning and mother housekeeping, each family in a home of its own) is held out to be both the normal way of living and the happiest place to be' (p. 241). The family was to fulfil two main functions: to socialize children and to provide a stable environment to which men can return from the alienating occupational world outside (Barrett 1988). Both these functions were mainly to be carried out by the wife and mother.

The family

The term 'family' was not always used in such a limited fashion. In 1869 the dictionary defined the term family as a number of different lifestyles (Barrett 1988). This included today's most common use of the term: 'persons of the same blood living under the same roof, and more especially the father, the mother and the children' (Barrett 1988: 201). However, it also included the use of the term for a set of kinsfolk who did not actually live together or an assemblage of co-residents who were not necessarily linked by blood or marriage. Barrett (1988) concluded: 'It is clear then, that when we speak of the family we should take care to distinguish what it is that we are referring to: an aggregation of kinsfolk or a household of co-residents' (p. 201).

The structure of the family is continually changing (Gavron 1968; Dennis and Erdos 1993). Today, people tend to make a variety of different lifestyle choices that are coherent with new family structures (Davies *et al.* 1993). For example, in the past the decisions to marry and to have children were made in consecutive order. Today they are increasingly viewed as two separate decisions. People who decide to have children do not necessarily decide to get married. People who get married do not necessarily decide to have children. About 25 per cent of couples are opting not to have children at all (McGoldrick 1989). Gay and lesbian couples decide to have children. People make conscious decisions to become single parent families.

In order to define today's structure of the family, it is important to consider the following recent trends. In only 16 per cent of American families do father, mother and children actually live together, 7% of children live in stepfamilies, 23% of children live in single mother families, 3% of children live in single father families (Phares 1992). In Britain today, one in eight adults with dependent children is a single parent (Hanmer and Statham 1988). Eighty per cent of all single mothers are divorced (not unmarried, as many presume) (McGoldrick 1989). In Northern Ireland, only 7.2% of all households conform to the typical image of the nuclear family (McShane and Pinkerton 1986).

Clearly, many children do not actually live with both their biological parents. However, Phares (1992) found that most of them have contact with their parents. In her study, 42 per cent of the children living with their mother had some contact with their father; for 19 per cent, this contact was weekly; 35 per cent had no contact with their biological father; 54 per cent of the children who were living with their biological father had some contact with their mother, 19 per cent had no contact with her. Children growing up in one-parent or step-parent families do not lose touch with their biological parents. The role of parents and their relationships to children has changed.

Changing family patterns

Some people argue that these changes are to the detriment of children and affect society as a whole negatively. Increasingly, single parents are blamed for growing crime rates, youth delinquency, homelessness, poor school attendance or low achievement. Research shows that growing up in a single parent or step-parent family does not automatically lead to problems (Schorr and Schorr 1989). It is not the structure of the family that is detrimental to children. Children adjust remarkably well to changing relationships provided that the adults around them can cope. The damaging factors are to be found in pressures put on the adult, the single parent.

Poverty and deprivation are the main stress factors for single parents (Schorr and Schorr 1989). The majority of single parents live on an income far below average and are socially isolated (Evason 1980a). In an attempt to prevent single parents from living in poverty and having to claim social benefits the British government established the so-called Child Support Agency (CSA) in 1993. The aim of this agency was to locate absent parents and ensure that they pay adequate maintenance to their children. Since its establishment the CSA has been heavily criticized. The role of the CSA in childcare work will be discussed further in Chapters 5 and 11. For now it is sufficient to say that women's groups claim that money collected from absent fathers is used to pay or replace benefits rather than increasing the money available to single mothers, thus saving the government millions of pounds. Single mothers and their children are no better off than they were before the establishment of the agency. In fact, many of them are worse off. In some cases ex-husbands deny fathering their own children in order to avoid payment. The effect of this on the children and their mothers is detrimental. Support groups of absent fathers have been formed. They claim that the financial demands for their first family leaves them and their second families in poverty. There is a backlog of thousands of cases waiting to be dealt with. A major review of the agency is in process.

Evason (1980b) criticized society 13 years earlier for not caring for single mothers adequately: 'The problems often flow from the failure of our society to cater for and adjust to the existence of such families' (p. 88). The situation for single mothers in Britain has not changed much. In some Scandinavian countries poverty prevention is institutionalized. Child maintenance is directly deducted from the absent father's salary (French 1993).

Oakley (1982) saw the problem from a feminist viewpoint:

> The position of women in single-parent families reveals particularly sharply the basic contours of the position of women in general. For the forces propelling female-headed single-parent families into poverty are the reasons why women in society as a whole do not have economic autonomy or equality with men. They can't earn enough to support themselves and their children – or they can't get jobs compatible with child rearing. (p. 293)

Concepts of the family

Historically speaking, changes in the structure of families should not come as a surprise. It is mistaken to think of 'the family' as a fixed entity. We discussed earlier how patterns of behaviour, relationships and roles change according to the situations in which people find themselves. This is a natural process. Developing concepts must be able to accommodate the nature of these changes. At first sight it may seem as if the trend towards a more flexible structure of the family would free women as well as men from rigid role expectations. This is not necessarily the case. In fact, role expectations remain and have led to much of the abuse of women in childcare work.

One of the reasons why childcare workers concentrate on mothers in their investigation and intervention can be found in the expectations of mothers' behaviour in relation to children. Mothers are, as Phares (1992) put it, 'expected to devote most or all their time to their children and therefore are seen the only culpable party when a child develops psychological problems' (p. 660). Mothers, in particular single mothers, generally spend much of their time looking after the welfare of their children. Many single mothers feel that they have to fulfil both a mother's and a father's role for their children. This means that they work particularly hard to achieve an environment that permits children to grow up into healthy and happy adults. Most of them succeed against the odds, despite the fact that the stakes are stacked against them.

An evolving concept of the family has to take changes in the structure of the family into account. Childcare workers are at the forefront of these changes. The majority of children on childcare workers' case loads grow up in single parent, mostly single mother, families. Childcare workers must be clear that the quality of relationships rather than the structure of the family is assessed.

Relationships outside the family

Women's roles and relationships within the family are tightly defined. There are clear expectations on how women are to behave in relation to men and children. Involuntary childlessness is viewed with pity, voluntary childlessness as an oddity (Hanmer and Statham 1988). Women who concentrate on relationships with other adults, be it in employment or leisure, are blamed when things go wrong within the family. Phares (1992) pointed out that:

> it appears that the nuclear family with mother working in the home and father working outside is still understood to be the norm and that employed mothers and unemployed fathers are seen as aberrant and blameworthy in the development of psycho-pathology in children and adolescents. (p. 661)

Employment

Employment helps to prevent poverty as well as social isolation. Sixty per cent of women in two-parent families are employed; 44.6 per cent of female-headed one-parent families depend on women's wages (Hanmer and Statham 1988). It has been estimated that the number of families in poverty would increase three-fold if women were not to contribute financially. However, as Hanmer and Statham (1988) pointed out 'work tends to be seen as paid, full-time, continuous, and outside the home' (p. 42). This concept does not reflect the experience of women. Women's employment is typically low paid, part-time, temporary and, at times, home-based.

In the late nineteenth century about one-quarter of British women were employed. Figures were similar for France and Italy (Scott and Tilly 1982). Working women were overwhelmingly members of the working and peasant classes, their jobs mainly in the domestic services, garment making or the textile industry (Scott and Tilly 1982). Today women from all social classes are working outside the home. While they occupy a much greater range of jobs, women workers still predominate in catering, cleaning, hairdressing and other personal services (75.6 per cent), clerical work (73.3 per cent), and education, welfare and health (64.8 per cent) (Oakley 1982). World-wide about 70–5 per cent of work is carried out by women. Yet, women earn only 10 per cent of the world's income and own only 1 per cent of the world's property (French 1993).

Recent Trends

Over recent years women's social mobility has been encouraged. The Fair Employment Commission has been set up for women who are discriminated against in appointments or promotion on gender grounds. Many employers today encourage equal opportunities for women. They explicitly encourage women applicants for higher level jobs. However, women are still vastly under-represented in these jobs and experience a 'glass ceiling' (French 1993) regarding promotion. In childcare work, women dominate the work force at basic levels. Yet, men typically predominate the profession higher up the occupational ladder (Hanmer and Statham 1988). As French (1993) put it, 'women [bear] most of the responsibility, while men [have] most of the power' (p. 31).

Job descriptions and demands of well paid, full-time, permanent high level jobs are not tailored to traditional expectations of women. Recently a drop in the numbers of women in these positions is therefore not surprising. These jobs were tailored for men. Managerial jobs are highly demanding and allow for little commitment outside of work. Traditional role divisions in the family freed men from household and childcare responsibilities and enabled them to take up demanding jobs. Employed women are still expected to do the lion's share of household and childcare duties when they return home from work (Gordon 1990; French 1993). Combining employment, parenthood and the running of a home is a formidable task. Support from employers cannot be expected. Severe lack of childcare facilities, restricted job choice and low wages mean that women enter employment with 'one hand tied behind their backs' (Cockburn 1982, in Gordon 1990: 8).

Leisure

Relationships with other adults, friendships and leisure activities are extremely important in the development and maintenance of social support networks outside the family for men as well as women. Women tend to have little time for leisure activities. This is not so for men. In most cultures men tend to engage in a range of hobbies or sports. French (1993) found employed as well as unemployed men playing games, frequenting pubs or just standing in groups in the streets during normal working hours. In many families weekends and evenings are predominated by men's sports interests. For example, when football is on the television nobody can watch anything else. When men are absent at weekends and evenings due to sports activities or visits to the pub women are left at home alone to mind the children.

For women too friendships are an invaluable resource. Women's friendships tend to be close and last for a long time (McGoldrick 1989). However, women are often forced to neglect their relationships with female friends during early adulthood, when their lives become preoccupied by family and young children (McGoldrick 1989). Most women clients and women childcare workers are in this situation. After fulfilling domestic as well as labour market demands women have neither the energy nor the time to engage in leisure or sports. This leads to isolation, lack of physical fitness and social outlets (Hanmer and Statham 1988).

Women's social relationships with adults outside the family is all too often considered of secondary importance to family needs. McGoldrick (1989) observed 'women have always played a central role in families, but the idea that they have a life cycle apart from their roles as wife and mother is a relatively recent one, and is still not widely accepted in our culture' (p. 29). Given the importance of friendships and their value for social support, it is important that childcare workers encourage clients to maintain friendships with other women. Childcare workers can help clients form new friendships by inviting them to take part in various groups, educational or leisure activities. During educational, sports or leisure activities women can meet with other women and form friendships. This is an important resource. Single mothers as well as women who live with men should be encouraged to ensure that they do not become socially isolated. Women need to learn to assert their need to have relationships and to socialize with other adults.

Conclusion

McGoldrick (1989) summarized in one sentence the essence of this chapter: 'We believe that the patriarchal system that has characterised our culture has impoverished both women and men' (p. 64). Women workers as well as clients are expected to fulfil roles in relation to their partners, children and other adults. Women's roles are clearly defined and limited. The main role of women is that of carer for men, children and the sick. Therefore, women are targeted by childcare services for investigation or intervention.

While the structures of marriage, family and labour market are changing, expectations of women's behaviour remain the same. Women's main duty is seen to be to her husband and her children. Employed women are still expected to do the full range of household chores when they get home from work. Lack of support facilities means that single mothers are unable to combine childcare and employment.

Women clients and women workers have much of this in common. Mothers are targeted by childcare workers because traditional role expectations cast them in the role of the main carer of children. Women childcare workers are cast in the same mould. In both cases women's behaviour is determined by traditional role expectations. These expectations are mainly determined by men. Many women are so strongly socialized into their roles that they no longer see the cast that moulded them. The traditional role of women in society has been so well established that over centuries women have learnt to accept it and behave accordingly. Attempts to break the mould have had little impact so far. Changes are slow.

Childcare workers are influenced by societal norms. They cannot ignore them. However, childcare workers are professionals. They are expected to transcend popular beliefs and lay wisdom. They are expected to base their practice on scientifically proven, theoretical frameworks. During the past century social scientists have looked at different aspects of human behaviour in society. Theories about the causes of this behaviour have flourished. The next chapter will look at the impact of theory on childcare work.

4

The role of theory in childcare work

Introduction

The previous chapter concentrated on traditional roles of women in society. Traditions are changing. Today women's lives are determined by changing family structures, changing relationship patterns and changing demands in employment. However, women are still the main target of childcare workers when there are problems with their children. They are still abused within the childcare system. The question remains as to why women are abused within this system. As trained professionals childcare workers should be sensitive to changes in societal norms and should encourage changes which benefit women. They realize the importance of empowering clients, and their role is often one of advocacy (Pinkerton 1994). Childcare courses today aim to provide sound theoretical grounding for practice. As Howe (1987) pointed out 'the utility of theory in modern science is to summarise existing knowledge, to categorise and relate observations, and to predict the occurrence of as yet unobserved events and relationships' (p. 12). Childcare workers are expected to integrate theory into their practice and to base their professional conduct on knowledge gained from professional courses.

In this chapter we will look at some of the theories which are taught in childcare courses and which, therefore, should form the basis of intervention for childcare workers. There are numerous theories, and, different courses emphasize different theories. For the purpose of this chapter, we will group together some of the main theories. This overview is by no means comprehensive. Theories discussed here are chosen because they influence the conduct of childcare workers especially in relation to their work with mothers and children. Psychodynamic theory, cognitive theory, theories of social development, as well as systems theory and feminist theory will be addressed in this context.

Most of these theories are helpful in providing a framework for childcare workers. However, we argue that they are generally insensitive towards the abuse of women in childcare work mainly because they are outdated. They do not take the changes described in the previous chapter into account. In fact, they perpetuate discrimination against women by a continued emphasis upon women as the main carer of children. Consequently, childcare workers hold women responsible when childcare or child protection problems arise. These theories give the impression that there is a scientific basis to such practice. Adherence to traditional role expectations is one reason why women are targeted in childcare work, outdated theories another.

Theoretical framework for childcare

Childcare practitioners are increasingly searching for sound theoretical frameworks on which to base their intervention. Psychodynamic theories (Erikson 1963; Strachney 1963), cognitive approaches (Piaget 1954; Beck 1976), theories of social development, attachment and loss (Bowlby 1969, 1973) as well as systems theory (Minuchin 1974; O'Hagan 1986) have all had an impact over the years. On the whole theories have informed and improved practice. However, many of the most popular theories in childcare work have not been sensitive towards women's issues. So far, they have not been able to prevent the abuse of women in childcare work. Theories in childcare are usually based on observations of child or parent behaviours or their interactions. The previous chapter showed that much of the behaviour of mothers and fathers stems from traditional role expectations. Women's behaviour in relation to their partners, their children and other adults is learnt. Past experiences shape each woman's behavioural repertoire and present contexts determine the actual performance. Cultural differences occur.

Childcare researchers either observe behaviours or apply questionnaires. In doing this they wittingly or unwittingly perpetuate the *status quo* by portraying the observed behaviour as inevitable or desirable. They then derive their theories from these observations, in the cultural context of their times. In most cases they do not concentrate on the way the behaviours in question have been learnt, but derive theoretical explanations from hypothetical cognitive structures or schemata: 'The emphasis is not on the child's behavior but on inferred surrogates of the behavior, called *interpretations* or *recognitions*, the only evidence of which is the very behaviors they are said to explain' (Schlinger 1992: 1405). Consequently, childcare workers base their practice on hypothetical constructs rather than actual behaviour. As Howe (1987) so aptly put it: 'What is to be done depends on what it is you think is going on' (p. 8). A full critical analysis of the process of theory formation goes beyond the realms of this book (for a detailed discussion, see Baum 1994). However, it is important to realize at this point that theories are formulated by people and therefore have to be viewed in cultural and historical contexts: 'For different people, the world around just looks different – physically, psychologically and socially' (Howe 1987: 8). Personal experiences and cultural context inevitably become part of the theory. Four main theories will now be addressed and their relevance to childcare work identified.

Psychodynamic theory

Sigmund Freud (1856–1939) was the founding father of psychodynamic theory. He developed his approach while treating mainly female patients, most of whom were seeking therapy for hysteria and other related nervous conditions. In Staats's (1994) words, 'Freud studied the verbalisations of neurotic patients in psychoanalysis' (p. 94). Freud then formulated his theory from this specialized area of psychology. He proposed that human behaviour was caused and determined by mental processes. He suggested that many of these mental processes remained in the unconscious (Smith 1990). He suggested that there were three 'force fields' to the human personality. The *id*, which he considered to be the 'biological bedrock of motivation', the *ego* which he thought to be responsible for 'adaptation to external reality' and the *superego* which he thought evoked 'feelings of guilt when values are broken' (Smith 1990: 20–1). Freud suggested that conflicts between these three fields lay at the bottom of psychological disturbance and that these conflicts developed during childhood.

Psychodynamic theory of child development

Freud constructed a theory of child development based on observations of his women patients. He identified complex structures of bizarre fantasies and anxieties, interrelated emotions and aspirations in his patients. He named these 'Oedipus complex' (Smith 1990). Freud chose the Greek story of Oedipus, son of King Laius and Queen Jocasta, because he felt that it captured two main themes of erotic fantasies: incest and patricide. He suggested that the so-called 'Oedipus complex' originated in childhood.

Most psychological theorists today agree that many adult behaviours stem from childhood experiences. Freud, however, took this assertion one step further when he suggested that many of the problems encountered by adults originated in children's erotic drives. The difference between adult and child eroticism, he suggested, was that children's erotic feelings were not aimed at sexual intercourse and that they were incestuous.

Psychodynamic theory and childcare work

There are obvious problems with psychodynamic theory when applied to childcare work. Freud's idea about children's erotic yearnings and incestuous feelings can all to easily be used to justify child sex abuse and excuse the perpetrator. Abusers as well as judges in abuse cases have based their statements and their judgements on such ideas when they stated that the child enticed the abuser and thus invited the abuse. Professionals working with child sex abuse have discovered clear patterns by which perpetrators shape the behaviour of the abused child. The perpetrator teaches the child behaviours which are concurrent with abuse but prevent disclosure. This process is best captured in the phrase 'grooming the child' (Furniss 1991).

Freud had also suggested that boys generally fear for their genitalia and that girls envy boys for having a penis. He called the two notions 'castration anxiety' and 'penis envy'. Stockard and Johnson (1980) captured today's assessment of these assertions when they wrote: 'Freud's idea that females are mutilated males and that females deeply envy males' genitalia is obviously sexist and unsupported by evidence' (p. 207). The idea of penis envy in the female child 'simply recognises the social fact that males really do have power' (p. 210).

Psychodynamic theory today

Freudian theory has to be viewed in the cultural context in which it was written. Women's lives in the late nineteenth and early twentieth century were considerably different from women's lives today (Chapter 3). An example of cultural differences at the turn of the century is the fact that Freud had formulated most of his theories before women in Britain finally attained the right to vote in 1918 (Scott and Tilly 1982). Freud's theory was based on observations within his cultural context. To give them validity today is clearly a distortion of the reality of women's lives at the end of the twentieth century.

Today, fundamental disagreements have split the psychodynamic school of thought, and it has become heterogeneous. Some theorists and therapists have continued in a classic Freudian tradition (Smith 1990), others have developed their own psychodynamic approaches, such as the Jungian approach (Carvalho 1990), or the Kleinian approach (Cooper 1990). Erikson's (1963) theory of life-span development is one of the most prominent neo-Freudian approaches in childcare work.

Erikson's life-span theory

Erikson (1963) was a careful observer of human behaviour and his theories are formulated in a way that is easily followed by the majority of childcare students. He used many of Freud's ideas about child development and extended them into a life-span approach. He postulated a range of psychosocial stages throughout the human life cycle. Erikson suggested that each of the stages represented a conflict between two poles (for example trust versus mistrust, initiative versus guilt, competence versus inferiority, intimacy versus isolation, egocentricity versus despair, etc.) and that each of these conflicts had to be resolved before the person can successfully proceed into the next stage.

Eriksonian theory and childcare work

There are at least three problems with Erikson's theory for childcare workers. First, Erikson used observations of behaviour to make inferences about mental states. This is a common practice of theorists and lay people alike. It inevitably leads to a circularity of the argument and modern thinkers aim to avoid it (Baum 1994). Second, his theory has strong inbuilt value systems. Words such as 'mistrust', 'guilt', 'inferiority', 'isolation', or 'despair' clearly indicate the preferred direction of development. People who do not resolve conflicts in this direction are seen to have problems. Third, Eriksonian theory does not offer a basis for intervention. Assessments, according to Erikson, lead to a dead-end. Take for example the notion that between birth and the age of one-and-a-half the child has to resolve the conflict between trust versus mistrust. A child can be assessed as mistrustful during this age; in other words, a child may behave in ways which can be described as mistrustful. However, mistrust does not explain the behaviour; the circumstances that lead to the behaviour do. For example, if the child was abused or neglected he/she was likely to develop behaviours that fit the description. The problem that requires intervention is not mistrust but the abuse or neglect.

Cognitive theory

Cognitive theories have had a widespread influence on social and health care professionals (Beck 1976). Childcare workers have obviously concentrated on theories of cognitive development. The ideas of the Swiss psychologist Jean Piaget (1954) have been in the forefront in this area and have shaped the conduct of childcare professionals for many decades. Piaget developed theories of cognitive as well as moral development based on observations of children's responses to certain experimental tasks (Staats 1994). Piaget believed that in order to understand why people behave the way they do we have to find out what they think, expect and know. He saw cognitive events as unique, separate from observable behaviour, possibly even causing such behaviour. He suggested that children integrate new experiences either by assimilation (adding cognitive concepts) or accommodation (changing existing cognitive concepts).

Cognitive theory and childcare work

Piaget's theory has been widely influential in childcare work. It has, however, been criticized from a number of directions. First, Piaget did not always define his terms operationally. It is, therefore, difficult for others to interpret his findings and his generalizations or repeat his experiments. Second, many of his studies lack proper controls, because he did not identify cause-and-effect relations between the variables. Third, Piaget presumed that children understood the words he used in his studies in the same way adults do. It is obvious that this is not the case. Children have to learn the meaning and the appropriate use of words before they can be tested on them.

The main problem with cognitive approaches is that in the search for an explanation of their observations cognitivists postulate that there are mental events or cognitive structures which caused the behaviour. Mental events or cognitive structures cannot have explanatory power because they are inferred from observations of the behaviour to be explained. They are hypothetical. Cognitivists believe that they have found an explanation for behaviour in these hypotheses. We will discuss the problems with this kind of misconception – that is, mentalistic analysis – in greater detail in Chapter 10. For now it is sufficient to say that making hypothetical inferences leads to abuse of women, because it leads childcare workers to conclude that the cause of child abuse or neglect lies in the cognitive structures of the adult, in most cases the mother. These inferences cannot be proven but wrongfully leave the impression that an explanation is found. Childcare workers who use this kind of analysis often look no further. They will not be able to identify the actual causes of abusive or neglectful behaviour such as the past or present experiences of the mother or the circumstances in which she is bringing up the children. Cognitive theories are, therefore, not sensitive to the actual reality of children's or of women's lives.

Theories of social development

There are, however, some theories that emphasize social and environmental influences on child behaviour. These are theories of social development, particularly those that emphasize attachment behaviours, reactions to loss or other social interactions. Theorists in these areas were usually keen observers of child behaviour and concentrate their efforts on the interactions between children and adults. Many of these observations yielded interesting results and fostered the development of increasingly sophisticated methods of observation (Carlson 1990). Theories formulated by Bowlby (1969, 1973) were highly influential in this area. He concentrated particularly on attachment behaviours and reactions to loss. Bowlby focused his work on the influence of the mother's behaviour on the child. He concluded that the mother was the most important person in the early part of an infant's life. He coined the term 'maternal bonding' to describe this relationship. Furthermore, he observed children's reactions to loss of mother and called these responses 'maternal deprivation'.

Mother-oriented theories

Bowlby was clearly of the opinion that the mother was to be the nourisher and main carer for young children and that it was her responsibility to provide good 'mothering'. He stated that

> what is ... essential for mental health is that the infant and young child should experience a warm, intimate and continuous relationship with his mother ... The evidence is now such that it leaves no room for doubt ... that the prolonged deprivation of the young child of maternal care may have grave and far-reaching effects on his character and so on the whole of his future life. (in Oakley 1982: 215)

Bowlby argued that the mother's more or less continual presence was necessary to ensure children's mental health. He identified three categories of maternal deprivation: (1) living with a mother who has an 'unfavourable' attitude to her child; (2) losing one's mother through death, illness or desertion; and (3) being removed from one's mother to strangers by medical or social agencies. Bowlby saw the main causes of maternal deprivation as illegitimacy, divorce, chronic parental illness or psychopathy, poverty, parental imprisonment, and maternal employment. He stated that 'any family suffering from one or more of these conditions must be regarded as a potential source of deprived children' (in Oakley 1982: 215).

Mother-oriented theories and childcare work

One of the main problems with Bowlby's theory is the fact that he focused mainly on the influence of the mother, rather than all adults involved with the child. The assumption that the mother is the most important person in the early part of an infant's life is based on the historical role definition of women described in the previous chapter and obviously sexist. Terms such as 'maternal bonding' or 'maternal deprivation' are based on an outdated, traditional world-view. Clearly, the arrangements that Bowlby described as ideal and necessary for healthy development are a far cry from present family realities.

Margaret Mead (1966, in Oakley 1982) observed: 'an exclusive and continuous relationship between mother and infant is only possible under highly artificial urban conditions' (p. 216). Furthermore, Mead was concerned that theories of maternal deprivation were 'a new and subtle form of anti-feminism in which men ... – under the guise of exalting the importance of maternity – are tying women more tightly to their children than has been thought necessary since the invention of bottle-feeding and baby carriages' (in Oakley 1982: 216).

Bowlby's influence on childcare practice

Despite these problems Bowlby's influence on childcare work has not waned. His concepts of attachment are widely used by childcare and health professionals to measure attachment and make inferences about the quality of 'mothering' provided for children. Children who smile at their mother, cling to her and cuddle into her in threatening situations are said to be securely attached. The inference being that she is providing effective mothering. Atkinson *et al.* (1983) explain 'all babies become attached to the mother by the time they are 1 year old, but the quality of the attachment differs depending on the mother's responsiveness to the baby's needs' (p. 76). Consequently, if the child 'ignores' the mother, shows 'ambivalent behaviours', or 'squirms angrily to get down' after being picked up by the mother, the inference is that she provides ineffective mothering or even that she is rejecting the child. Atkinson *et al.* (1983) conclude that

> most babies show *secure attachment*, but some show *insecure attachment*. The avoidance or ambivalent behaviour shown by insecurely attached babies on reunion with the mother is assumed to be a defence against the anxiety occasioned by a mother who cannot be depended on ... Insecure attachment is associated with insensitive or unresponsive mothering during the first year of life. (p. 76)

Making such inferences from behavioural observations is dangerous. We addressed the dangers of making inferences from behavioural observations earlier. In this case inferences are used to label mother–infant relationships without taking full account of the circumstances in which they have evolved. We have addressed the complexities of relationships in the previous chapter. Assessments which are based on incomplete accounts of these complexities and instead make hypothetical inferences lead to judgemental childcare practices and consequently to the abuse of mothers in childcare work.

Learning appropriate attachment and separation behaviours

Children encounter numerous brief separations from their mothers, their fathers or others throughout the day and throughout their lives. For example, parents leave to go to work, spend time in another room or go out for the evening. There are ways to teach children separation behaviours which will help them deal with separation and loss without distress (Dillenburger and Keenan 1993). Some parents teach their children these types of appropriate separation behaviours at an early age. For example, children can be taught not to cry at separation but to adjust quickly to new situations (Gewirtz and Kurtines 1991). In these cases parents aim to equip their children with skills which are of benefit now and which will help the child adjust in later life. In traditional childcare assessments these parents and their children would be labelled as having formed avoidant attachments. More appropriately these parents should be assessed as having paid particular attention to what is best for their child.

The role of fathers in child development

Developmental theories mentioned above are restrictive, labelling and abusive towards women. However, they also affect men negatively. Fathers are often under-represented in research. The psychologist Vicky Phares (1992) has recently offered a review of empirical and theoretical child and adolescent literature to ascertain why compared with mothers, fathers are dramatically under-represented in clinical research literature. She found that

> the tendency to blame mothers for the psychological problems of their children has been well documented ... [and that] ... mother blaming has been described as a sexist bias towards studying mothers' contributions to child and adolescent maladjustment while at the same time ignoring similar contributions by fathers. (p. 656)

The only area where fathers are investigated to the exclusion of mothers is child sex abuse (Phares 1992). However, in most families fathers spend much time with their children and influence their development considerably. Assumptions that the influence of fathers is negligible reflect outdated beliefs about the role of men and women in child rearing. They perpetuate the kind of role restrictions for women described in the previous chapter. Phares concluded that 'excluding fathers from child and adolescent research is not warranted on the assumption of lack of time spent with their children. Overall research has shown that fathers influence their children in ways that are very similar to the ways that mothers do' (p. 657).

Developmental theories in childcare courses

Theories of social development based on one sided, mother oriented observations are still taught in many training courses for childcare workers. They are also prevalent in the 'mother and baby' literature so widely propagated on the lay person's market (Urwin 1985). This is happening despite vast differences between the role of women in the early part of this century, when many of these theories were first formulated, and the reality of women's lives at the end of the twentieth century. Gordon (1990) saw this discrepancy clearly.

> That children and homes are constructed and represented as the responsibility of women, is indicated in the debates about maternal deprivation and working mothers, where a mother at home is considered the normal situation; anything else is a deviation and a source for concern, research and speculation. (p. 15)

Theories in childcare work have to reflect the fact that 'anything else' is the norm at the end of the twentieth century, if they are to bear any resemblance to the reality of most children and families today.

Childcare practices today

Phares (1992) pointed out that today 'it cannot be assumed that mothers are the primary source of parental influence on children's psychological adjustment in all families' (p. 656). In fact, this is not only true for modern families. Historically children were looked after by a great number of people, for example grandmothers, aunts, siblings or nannies. Today the number of people looking after a child is probably smaller than in past extended families. However, while 60 per cent of women with children under the age of 18 are in the work force the idea that only one person, the mother, should look after a child is wholly unrealistic.

The essential issues for healthy and well adjusted child development are neither the gender of the carer nor the structure of the family. Essential is the level of love, stimulation, guidance and stability provided. For example, Phares (1992) pointed out that 'there is evidence that, beginning in infancy, infants show very similar patterns of attachment to their mothers and fathers, which appears to be due to concordant parenting styles within parental dyads' (p. 657). Consistent parenting rather then 'mothering' is the key to healthy child development.

Systems theory

One theory which on the surface seems to have taken account of the role of father and mother in childcare work is systems theory. Over the past decade systems theory has evolved as one of the main social and health care theories (O'Hagan 1986). In brief, systems theory provides a framework in which the individual is viewed within the context of social systems, such as the family, the neighbourhood network, the community, etc. Systems theory proposes that the system is larger than the sum of its parts. Within each large system, theoretical subsystems are constructed, such as sibling subsystems or parental subsystems in the larger system of the family, pressure group subsystems in the larger system of the community, etc. Conceptually, each system and each subsystem has boundaries. Boundaries are considered to be either rigid or permeable (Minuchin 1974).

Systems theory and childcare work

As a framework for childcare workers, systems theory has offered helpful concepts. Other theories viewed the individual in relative isolation. Individual case work was based on such approaches. The presenting problem was located inside the individual. Systems theory views people and their problems in their social context. The presenting problem is viewed as a problem of the whole family, a problem of their interactions. Individuals are viewed as bound into a system of relationships. Treatment of problems is aimed at changing the system rather than the individual (Minuchin and Fishman 1981). Childcare workers who operate within a systems framework usually gain a contextual, holistic view of client problems (Walround-Skinner 1976). However, systems theory has not been beyond criticism. McGoldrick (1989) pointed out that systems theory takes incomplete account of the reality of women's lives. It can be 'gender biased' and lead to 'male derived, male-focused ideas about behaviour and relationships' (p. 62).

Feminist theory in childcare work

The only area where female-derived and female-focused ideas are dominant in childcare work is feminist theory (Oakley 1982; Barrett 1988; Gordon 1990). Feminist theories focus on gender-related inequality, discrimination and oppression and usually aim to achieve women's equality and empowerment in many areas of women's lives. Howe (1987) stated optimistically that 'conceived in the seventies, born in the eighties, feminist theory and practice is set to develop into a major social work perspective' (p. 125). Today, in the mid-1990s this aim has not been fully achieved. Feminist theories have alerted childcare workers to many important issues related to the role of women in childcare work; for example, the oppression of women (Langan and Day 1992), violence perpetrated against women (Hanmer and Maynard 1987) and the importance of woman-centred practice (Hanmer and Statham 1988). However, as discussed in Chapter 2, feminist thinking seems to have had limited impact on the daily conduct of most childcare workers. Clearly, feminist theories have not yet been able to prevent the abuse of women in childcare work.

Why have feminist theories not been able to protect women and prevent the abuse of women in childcare work? One reason may be that these theories have not been sensitive enough to detect the subtleties of the abuse of women in childcare work. Another reason may be that these theories were formulated by women. Ramazanoglu (1987) identified male-dominated hierarchies in academia and pointed out that these structures will act to subordinate female academics. Some feminist theories have over compensated for this imbalance. They have been criticized for being extreme or even 'men-hating' (Hudson 1993). Clearly, this cannot be the aim of theories which promote equality. It seems so far that in many areas of childcare work the impact of feminist theories and 'the acceptance of the relevance of issues of gender remained tokenistic' (Hudson 1993: 137).

The emerging picture

Most childcare theories still view parenting as a mainly female domain. Assumptions based on such concepts, for example, 'maternal bonding', lead to mother blaming. Practice as well as research based on such assumption do a disservice to women and men alike. It has been noted 'that before the mid-1970s, fathers were not included in child development research because the cultural norm dictated that the father's role was to provide for the family financially, and it was considered unmasculine for men to be involved in taking care of the children' (Phares 1992: 659). This is no longer the case.

The roles of men and women have changed. The traditional image of the family is no longer reality. Today nearly one-half of all marriages end in divorce, the highest rate in history. People decide to get married later (average age at marriage is 25 years) than ever before (records begun in 1890). Many couples (2 million) decide to live together rather than get married. This figure is four times higher than it was in 1960. More than 10 per cent of adults live alone and over 16 million children live with only one or neither parent (Zimbardo 1988). Looking at these figures it becomes clear that the majority of people do not live in a traditional two-parent family. It can no longer be presumed that women are supported by a male breadwinner or that they are available to look after the children of the family. New family structures are evolving. Fathers as well as relatives, friends, neighbours, child minders, crèche facilities or nurseries are increasingly involved in the rearing of children. Childcare theories must take account of these changes.

Conclusion

Traditional theories are still prominent in the work of childcare workers today. The majority of courses for childcare workers base their teaching on these theories and encourage childcare workers to integrate them into their practice. In this chapter we looked at psychodynamic theory, cognitive theory, theories of social development, attachment and loss as well as systems theory and feminist influences. Many of these theories have been widely criticized and are outdated. Some have a clear gender bias and are directly mother oriented. Systems theory as well as feminist theories have had promising influences in counterbalancing this state of affairs; however, they too have not been able to eradicate the abuse of women in childcare work. A new approach is clearly needed and will be introduced in Part III of this book.

The next two chapters will look at the impact of the whole childcare system on women. Childcare workers do not work in isolation. They are bound into a system of ideologies, convictions and popular beliefs, policies, procedures and laws. The system, while aimed at the protection of children and families, is in fact often abusive towards mothers. Childcare workers operate within an abusive childcare system.

5

Abusive childcare systems I

Introduction

Chapter 2 explored apparent 'safeguards' against recently exposed abuse of women by childcare professionals, and found them ineffective. Much of the fundamental social, structural and theoretical underpinning of that abuse was considered in Chapters 3 and 4. This chapter will explore more immediate contributory factors. There are many of them; for example, the prevailing political climate (such as, the government's current thinking on single mothers) is very abusive in its manifestations and long-term effects. Each of these factors can function as a significant part of what has become known (and, more importantly, experienced by parents) as a 'system of abuse' or the 'abusive childcare system'. This chapter will begin by asking what is meant by 'system'. It will differentiate between the traditional meaning of 'system' and the derogatory meaning given to it by parents who have been intentionally and/or unintentionally abused by childcare professionals. It will then ask why women are much more likely than men, or couples, to be abused by such systems. A detailed exploration of each of the potentially abusive factors within these systems will follow, with reference to research, childcare literature and experience.

The meaning of 'system'

In research on parental participation in child protection work (O'Hagan 1994b), the most common critical utterance by parents questioned (many of whom were single mothers) was: 'you can't beat the system'; Hooper (1992) speaks of mothers' distress 'channelled into fighting the system

to regain their children' (p. 157). Childcare professionals hear this exasper-
ated cry by parents again and again in their daily work. Professionals
themselves, and writers on child protection, often use the term disparag-
ingly. Milner (1993) writes of the child protection *system* 'acting as yet
another distant father, scrutinizing social workers scrutinizing mothers
already under enormous pressures' (p. 59). Hearn (1990) believes in an
all-embracing system in which the government, through structural and
legislative mechanisms, increases 'men's power over and oppression of
women' (p. 68).

But what do parents mean by the 'system'? What do the public
commonly mean by 'system'? The *Shorter Oxford Dictionary* (Little *et al.*
1983) defines 'system' as:

> an organized or connected group of objects; a set or assemblage of
> things connected, associated, or interdependent, so as to form a
> complex unity; a whole composed of parts in orderly arrangement
> according to some scheme or plan; [it is] rarely applied to a simple or
> small assemblage of things.

This definition has resonance in the reason why many social work theorists
from diverse professional and ideological stances have propounded
systems theory as a sound underpinning for family and childcare work (for
example, Janchill 1969; Walrond-Skinner 1976; O'Hagan 1986). But it is
an inadequate definition for understanding and identifying aspects of
childcare work which parents, particularly mothers, have experienced as
abusive. The abusive attitudes and behaviour of some childcare professionals are not necessarily 'organized', 'connected', 'associated' or
'interdependent' as in the dictionary definition of system; parents and
children may perceive them to be so, but often they are independent,
unassociated and unconnected, their manifestations predictable and
unpredictable, regular or intermittent, singular or multiple. More importantly, their manifestations are unlikely to be intentional: childcare
professionals do not deliberately abuse women, and very often are
unaware when they are doing so.

In identifying abusive childcare systems, three questions arise: *what*
precisely are the abusive components of such systems? *who* are the
abusers? and *why* do they abuse (motivation)? The answer to the first
question is that there are many abusive components and contributory
factors within childcare systems. Here are a few of them: the prevailing
political climate is distinctly hostile towards single mothers, and the words
and actions of senior politicians are intensifying their isolation and stigma.
Politicians may also exploit public opinion on a range of child-related
issues, and formulate childcare laws leading to potentially abusive childcare policies and procedures. Away from the political sphere, the actions of
childcare professionals may stem from common beliefs which are abusive

of women, or, equally abusive convictions based upon personal experiences, rather than upon professional criteria. The answer to the second question is that social workers, police, health visitors, paediatricians, community nurses, psychiatrists, teachers, DSS officers, and, the managers of any of these agencies are all capable of abusing women, directly or indirectly, unintentionally or intentionally (the latter being extremely rare, though the chapter contains one example of this). Third, their motivations are many and varied; they may include blatant sexism and racism, or fear, or a preoccupation with risk (due to some near-miss fatality in the past). We will explore these and many more motivating factors in more detail.

Women: frontline victims facing frontline workers?

Why the abuse of women? Do childcare systems not abuse men equally so? There is no reliable research on the matter, but there are numerous reasons (see Chapters 3 and 4) for thinking the answer is 'no'. Generally, the traditional role women play as mothers, wives and carers guarantees they will be engaged by a whole array of welfare professionals, infinitely more so than men (Brook and Davis 1985). More specifically, as the principal carers of children, the vast majority of parents in contact with childcare professionals, are women. Milner (1993) with some justification, considers the term 'parenting' in much childcare literature an 'empty gesture', as invariably in childcare work, it is referring to the responsibilities undertaken by mothers who are always easily accessible, and abrogated by fathers who are largely inaccessible. This accessibility of mothers is most clearly seen in medical childcare services. These services have made great technological and medical progresses in many aspects of childcare, primarily because of the accessibility of mothers and mothers-to-be, and their willingness to be seen, supervised, monitored, directed and researched by a host of medical and childcare professionals. Fathers have remained invisible to, or, invariably regarded as irrelevant, by medical personnel. Miles (1991) writes of the medicalization of childcare and the resulting wider surveillance of child health (meaning of course the surveillance of mothers).

Men and women can both be abused by particular components of childcare systems. But mothers remain so overwhelmingly at the frontline in childcare, that the risk of them being abused is infinitely greater. More important, many of the specifically women-abusive components have become so entrenched within childcare systems, so influential and pervasive, that they cannot easily be eradicated. But they can and must be explored.

Exploring the principal components and processes of abusive childcare systems

---

The 'political flavour of the day'

Few areas of professional activity can match childcare in its vulnerability to the ideology of politicians. Statham's (1987) study of 'the new right' charts the disastrous impact of Thatcherism upon welfare generally. King and Trowell (1992) point out the rapid change of emphasis for childcare social work which took place during the Thatcher years, when social workers, influenced and pressurized by a harsh new climate of decisiveness and urgency, in which risk was not to be tolerated, increasingly became like police officers and surveillance operators, and when preventive childcare work fell by the wayside. As the following examples will demonstrate, however, ideology is not the only motivator in politicians' attempts to influence childcare; political opportunism may also be a factor, generating a climate of opinion which is potentially and actually abusive towards the principal carers of children.

1 Single parent mothers The Finer (1974) report revealed the poverty, stigma, and childrearing difficulties of one parent families, 90 per cent of whom were women. It demonstrated the urgent need for additional resources of childcare facilities to prevent a downward spiral leading to further family fragmentation and the removal of children. Politicians from all parties applauded the report and unanimously supported its recommendations. In doing so, they represented a public consciousness of the plight of many single parents and their children, exposed by such classics as the play *Cathy Come Home*. In this atmosphere of sympathy and moral consciousness, the government of the day initiated social and welfare reforms, the most radical of which was the Homeless Person's Act.

Few politicians mention Finer today; perhaps fewer are aware of its existence. The number of single parent mothers has increased three-fold since Finer; so too has their poverty and lack of opportunity. Politicians no longer talk about the problems faced by women singlehandedly rearing children; most politicians now speak of such mothers as the problem itself. Single parent mothers are generally perceived across the political spectrum as (1) an enormous drain on the country's resources; and (2) a threat to the social and moral fabric of society. This change in politicians' perceptions of single parents can be traced back to the early years of Thatcherism, but it was not until 1993 that the extent of their prejudice and resentment of single parent mothers became more boldly manifest, based as it was on their realization that the perceptions of both the public and the media, towards single parent mothers, had also changed dramatically. Thus Cabinet Minister John Redwood could refer to single parent mothers as 'one of the biggest social problems of the day' (*The Observer*, 1993), conveniently oblivious to the increasing number of unemployed, uneducated, of-no-fixed-address men, who floated about from single parent to single parent, fathering children whom they immediately made fatherless by deserting them. Television programmes previously noted for their no-holds-barred investigation of injustices against those too poor and vulnerable to defend themselves, inexplicably joined the anti-single parent mother crusade; for example, *Panorama* (BBC1, 1993) and *World In Action* (Granada Television, 1993) became the mouthpiece of Conservative politicians who saw the solution to the problem of single parent mothers in the harsh, punitive so-called 'corrective' programmes adopted by some American states. More extreme Conservative politicians argued for compulsory adoption of the children of single parent mothers.

The anti-single parent crusade became central in a so-called 'Back-to-Basics' philosophy promulgated at the Conservative Party annual conference in October, 1993. 'Principle', 'honour', 'loyalty', 'honesty', and 'personal responsibility' were terms frequently used to explain the philosophy; single parenthood was perceived as the very antithesis of such values; single parent mothers were unprincipled, promiscuous, irresponsible teenagers; they were gobbling up the biggest slice of the social security budget; they were rearing children who would inevitably turn to crime; they were exploiting the nation's scarce resources, particularly housing; they were becoming pregnant merely to jump the housing queue; etc. The Government, therefore, has repealed the Homeless Persons' Act. Homeless single parent mothers and their children are no longer regarded as the priority they once were under previous legislation; they are no longer guaranteed permanency of accommodation. Thus the probability that many mothers will have to move, again and again, and their children made to suffer the emotional and psychological effects of impermanency: continually changing homes, schools, communities and peer groups. This crusade against single parent mothers has been highly effective in stigmatizing and scapegoating them. Despite being exposed for its vindictiveness and hypocrisy (even in much of the Tory press), it succeeded in implanting in the public consciousness the dangerous conviction that single parent mothers were somehow to blame for the miseries endured by millions in a recession unparalleled in postwar Britain. It is not unlikely that some frontline childcare professionals have also been influenced by the crusade; have felt vindicated and supported in a more judgemental and unyielding attitude to single parent mothers; less empathic, more inclined to think in terms of caution and warning, and threats of removal if lifestyle does not change, if the standard of childcare does not dramatically improve. No one knows precisely how the crusade influenced and/or dictated the attitudes and practices of a whole host of agencies with whom single parent mothers and their children have contact.

2 Public outrage – political action – moral panic It is now common knowledge that local and national politicians and their civil servants over-reacted to the Maria Colwell tragedy (DHSS 1974) by formulating law, policies and procedures which had enormous potential for the abuse of mothers (interestingly, that abuse began with the Local Authority involved removing the last child of Maria's mother, long after the man convicted of her murder, Frank Kepple, was under lock and key – a clear example of a woman paying the ultimate price demanded by society for the crime of the man). The 1975 Children Act introduced necessary principles on children's rights, but it also led to increasingly insensitive and damaging child abuse investigations and interventions; and when interventions led to care proceedings and removal, parents were certain to have a much more difficult task in getting their children back again. The parent most likely to be in the frontline of that battle was the mother.

This increased state intervention, particularly the removal and fostering of children, was not universally in the children's interests; substantial research during the 1970s and 1980s demonstrates the abrupt, ill-prepared manner in which many children were removed from home, and drifted in and out of foster homes and residential homes (Rowe and Lambert 1973; Page and Clarke 1977; Kahan 1979; Millham *et al.* 1986; Triseliotis 1989; Kelly 1989). Single parent mothers bore the brunt of this vigorous interventionism. Many of them endured what they regarded as the unnecessary and unjustified removal of their children, and who then, during access, could see all the indicators of deterioration in their children's condition. Those who were frontline childcare workers during that period (including the authors) can recall the ceaseless flow of 'urgent' memos and updates of procedures quickly following on the publication of each report. This had nothing to do with child protection; it was merely the official stamp of approval for a far more self-protective, intrusive monitoring that greatly exacerbated the mother's predicament; but it was compatible with the atmosphere generated by politicians' responses to each tragedy, and their predictable reassurances to their constituencies: 'this cannot . . . must never happen again'. The Maria Colwell tragedy was the first of some 30 or more cases to generate a 'moral panic' among politicians, childcare managers and practitioners alike.

3 'Remove the children – how dare they remove the children!' Despite the more interventionist policies stemming from the 1975 Children Act, many more horrific deaths of children were revealed through court proceedings and public enquiries (DoH 1991a). Politicians and the media, therefore, remained generally critical of childcare professionals, particularly social workers. In 1986, however, public and political perceptions of childcare professionals substantially changed. Following the revelations of widespread sexual abuse of children and the crusade against it, childcare professionals (who figured prominently in the crusade) were increasingly perceived as the saviours of the victims of child sexual abuse. The anti-child sexual abuse crusade was supported by prominent entertainment and business personalities.

Political reaction to it was entirely predictable; most politicians, local and national, wanted to be part of it! Politicians of the day, including high profile Government ministers were fed statistics and advice now totally discredited (Goddard 1988; O'Hagan 1989; Howitt 1992). They appeared on radio and television shows discussing child sexual abuse; they wrote articles and gave comment to the press; they shared the experts' opinion that children allegedly sexually abused should be removed immediately and questions asked afterwards; they gave enthusiastic support to social workers and police officers doing the removals; they increased the considerable pressure they had already placed on social workers to remove children in the wake of many highly publicized deaths. But the Cleveland enquiry (Butler-Sloss 1988) report confirmed how little attention was given to the means of removal of children allegedly sexually abused, or to the impact on both child and primary carer, that is, the mother. Mothers, subjected to hamfisted investigative tactics leading to instant removal of their children, then denied access to and knowledge of their children's placements, were the principal victims in Cleveland.

As the tide turned, politicians swiftly turned too. They condemned 'overzealous' professionals, arrogant paediatricians and heavy handed police officers (all of these professionals had previously been the subject of politicians' praise and admiration). Yet when the suspicion arose of something perceived to be even more terrible than sexual abuse, namely, satanic and ritual abuse, some politicians behaved in precisely the same way again. They initially supported the removal of children in police-inspired dawn raids. Many single parent mothers faced those raids, and all their traumatic effects, alone. Two lone mothers in Orkney were the subject of particularly brutal raids (Black 1992).

Childcare principles perverted

The interpretation and application of childcare principles will determine both their moral and practical worth. Childcare is a minefield of moral and practice dilemmas, and childcare principles are vitally necessary as a pivotal support and guide for workers. But such principles are subject to an infinite number of interpretations, applications and exploitations, in an infinite variety of childcare situations. The moral and practice worth of principles can then be reduced substantially. Let us look at two of the most commonly known childcare principles: 'the welfare of the child is paramount', and, 'children need loving homes for which residential care is no substitute'.

1 The welfare of the child is paramount This is the central and most pervasive principle in childcare legislation, agency policy and procedure, and frontline practice. Many childcare professionals interpret the welfare principle as meaning nothing more than protecting the child from physical and sexual abuse, or neglect (O'Hagan 1989, 1993). But the 1989 Children Act has a far more profound and demanding meaning of 'welfare'; it means all aspects of the child's development, that is, emotional, psychological, physical, social and educational development. Removing a child because of the threat of harm or impediment to his/her physical development, without considering the impact of removal upon the child's welfare overall, is not in accord with the welfare principle. Ignoring any of the other vital aspects of development either during assessment or in preparation for removal, ensures not just that the child may suffer more, but that the primary carer, upon whom much of this development depends, will be similarly abused.

Unfortunately, this possibility is not always considered by those who think about the child's welfare only in the context of the child him/herself. Unlike King and Trowell (1992) who speak of the difficulty of separating the child as a unit of interest from the family of origin, there are many frontline childcare workers who not only have no such difficulty, but who automatically think and act as though there is a marked dichotomy between the welfare of the child and the rights of the mother. Worse still, there are some workers and childcare trainers who believe that the welfare of one is incompatible with the rights of the other, and, that their responsibility is to ensure the former by ignoring the latter. A distressed student recently attempted to voice her concerns about the impact of a particularly unprofessional, hasty, insensitive removal of a child, upon the mother of the child. The senior replied that the mother 'was of no concern to him'. Such workers are not likely to see any merit in Lawrence's (1992) perceptive feminist study; she states: 'The psychological welfare of children is inseparable from that of their mothers, and any notion of child protection needs to take account of this' (p. 32).

The severance of a child from a primary carer is emotionally painful and damaging to both; it is also psychologically damaging when a mother has to listen to the repetitive utterances of a principle (clearly misunderstood and misinterpreted), used to justify such actions; this is particularly so when the actions have been carried out insensitively (as they were in the case quoted above, and in Cleveland (Butler-Sloss 1988), Rochdale (Justice Brown 1991) and the Orkneys).

Mothers will hear of the welfare principle in interviews, case conferences, court hearings and reviews; it will be mentioned by all kinds of professionals. Often, the actions taken in pursuit of the principle are precisely the actions which those who formulated it, wanted childcare professionals to avoid; in which case, the principle becomes nothing more than a convenient platitudinous soundbite, impressing gullible lay people and professionals alike.

2 Residential homes are no fit place for children A single parent mother received a letter from the Social Services department, informing her that the residential home in which her son was placed was closing and that her son was to be placed with foster parents. She was told that her social worker would be contacting her to 'discuss' the matter, and in particular the contact that she would be allowed with her son. The mother was shocked and angry and contacted the social worker first. She had been well used to the residential home, the staff, the routine and the liberal hours of contact. The social worker attempted to reassure her that it was in her child's best interests. The mother could not be persuaded. Her scepticism was justified, as the number of contacts with her child were drastically reduced and the relationship with the foster parents deteriorated.

Much publicity has been given to the closure of psychiatric hospitals and the disastrous consequences for mentally ill people, many of whom have ended up in prison, on the streets, or dead (not to mention the number of innocent bystanders who have been injured by discharged mentally ill people). Less publicity had been given to a similar policy begun in the 1970s of closing children's residential homes, nor of the consequences for children and their primary carers. By 1986 one authority, Warwickshire, had decided to close every one of its children's homes. The roots of these two developments in health and social policy are similar: an ideological and principled stance that *all* residential care is inadequate at best and more often harmful. With regard to children, there was the additional factor of substantial research (to which we have already referred) demonstrating how badly children had suffered throughout the 1970s and 1980s by being abruptly removed and getting lost in the care system. Those senior managers who intended closing that system down were not interested in hearing about good quality residential care (Pick 1981), nor in research findings which verified the existence of such (SSI 1993), nor, least of all, about children who were more than satisfied in their residential homes (children in Leeds, for example, took Leeds City Council to court, because the authority decided to close their home without consulting them (Francis 1992)). There was another motivating factor: a naive conviction that high-quality, long-term fostering was readily available for all the children currently in the residential homes to be closed.

Contact between a mother and her child is made more difficult when the child is moved from a residential home to a long-term foster home. Few foster parents genuinely welcome natural parents, for obvious reasons; few natural parents find it easy to meet those judged to be more competent parents than themselves (O'Hagan 1993; Reder *et al.*, 1993). This, of course, is much less important than whether or not the child is being adequately cared for by foster parents. If it could be argued that the closure of residential homes, replaced by long-term fostering (and the consequential lessening of contact between child and parent), has proved to be beneficial to all children, to *all* aspects of children's welfare, then the closures (and the ideological antipathy towards residential homes upon which such a principle is based) would be universally welcomed and adopted. Regrettably, this is not the case, and the frequency of abuse in foster care (Benedict *et al.* 1994) demonstrates the naivity of those who simultaneously closed homes and weakened already tenuous contact between children and their natural families.

Abusive common beliefs

Common beliefs often motivate and direct the abuse of women in childcare work. The workers may not recognize them as such; on the contrary, they may believe them to be sound and tested theory. Tony Latham and his colleagues believed the notorious 'Pindown' was ethically and theoretically sound, based upon commonsensical ideas on human nature (Levy and Kahan 1991). Workers at all levels of childcare agencies are capable of similar misinterpretations. Others are well aware that it is their prejudices and convictions which are dictating their actions. Sommerfeld and Hughes (1987) researched the motivation of healthcare professionals (nurses, physicians and social workers) and discovered the majority disregarded professional criteria in favour of their subjective judgements. The following are examples of common beliefs manifest in such a way that they inevitably abuse women.

1 The collusive mother This belief promotes the suggestion that very large numbers of mothers are aware of abuses being perpetrated against their children and consciously decide not to do anything about it. There is nothing more formidible and threatening to a mother than being confronted with a group of professionals who do not believe her protestations of innocence, who are convinced that she knew and/or participated in the abuse, and that her principal objective is to protect the abuser at the expense of the child. This belief emerged forcibly in the 1980s, though its origins can be seen much earlier in writers such as Kempe and Kempe (1978). Many practitioners (including the authors of this text) and some researchers (for example Hooper 1992) have encountered mothers who have felt unable to inform agencies that their child was being abused; the main reason is the threat of violence from their partners and the fear of losing their children. There are undoubtedly some cases in which mothers have not informed agencies for more sinister reasons. To suggest however, that virtually every mother (as was suggested by Kempe) is colluding in, or consciously facilitating the regular abuse of their children, borders on a pathological perception of the mother and the mother–child relationship, and has no validity either in practice experience or credible research (Hooper (1992) and O'Hagan (1989) are two texts in particular which expose the paucity of logic in the belief).

An associated belief suggests that 'the alleged perpetrator and their accomplice' (usually regarded as mother) must admit that they abused the child, and that no progress can be made until they do so. Howitt (1992) refers to this as the 'contrition theory', equally lacking in research validity, though undoubtedly capable of inflicting additional abuse on mothers.

2 The all-coping, 'you'll manage it' mother Women are sometimes perceived by professionals as mothers capable of enduring extraordinary pressures and stresses. We have seen in earlier chapters that this perception has powerful cultural and historical roots. The mother's needs are consequentially subordinated to the needs of the child, even though fulfilling the needs of the child very much depends upon her (that is, the mother's) own needs being met. Parton (1990) takes issue with Dale *et al.* (1986) for their attitude to a young mother they had been helping; they decided she no longer needed the support of the Family Centre she had been attending, yet, 'there were times when she was extremely tired, times when she became irritable and depressed, and times when her relationships with Jeremy (the father of her child) became more stressful' (Dale *et al.* 1986: 152–3). Popay's (1992) research on the pervasive and chronic tiredness experienced by most women suggests that such tiredness is an illness induced by the organization imposed upon their lives and the social expectations of their roles: 'If chronic or severe tiredness is a persistent feature of fulfilling the mother and wife role then it is only to be expected that women will feel under pressure to cope with this too, and not to complain' (p. 117).

Stresses that bring mothers to the precipice of depression, despair and potential aggression towards their children, are often missed or ignored by professionals, and if mothers do go over the precipice they are made to feel that they have failed in some way. Women of differing ethnic origins may be more vulnerable to this kind of abuse. Afro-Caribbean women are perceived as mentally and physically stronger, their loyalty to their children and their ability to withstand all kinds of pressures and stresses, greater (Bryan 1991). The Afro-Caribbean extended family is often perceived as a most convenient safety net which will ensure that no young mother in its midst will sucumb.

3 Grandmothers know better Some professionals and their managers instinctively aim to enlist the support of the maternal grandmothers in childcare cases. Their instincts and their experiences tell them that grandmother is a far more mature, responsible, dependable and wise carer/person than the mother (another untested, unresearched belief which owes much to culture and history). Mothers are invariably seen as children themselves, especially if they are teenage mothers who have had deprivations and impairments in their own development (in 22 of the child abuse enquiry reports, mother's average age was 18.5 (Reder *et al.* 1993)). This perception of the mother being nothing other than a child in need of a mother is insulting and dangerous, yet shared by many childcare professionals and openly expressed in case conferences, reviews and in childcare proceedings. The very favourable attitude towards grandmothers was much in evidence in many of the child abuse enquiry reports (DHSS 1982; DoH 1991a) in which numerous young mothers alternated between their male partners (much to the anxiety of professionals) and their own mothers (always perceived by professionals as safer). A Health Visitor in the Lucy Gates tragedy (Bexley 1982) lamented that Lucy's mother 'needed a grandma figure 24 hours a day'. Sadly, many professionals do not seem to realize that their faith in grandmothers is very often unrealistic; worse, it can be a major source of abuse to the mother they're trying to help. It had disastrous consequences in the Tyra Henry case (Lambeth 1987) for both mother and child.

4 'Men are simply not worth bothering about' Many professionals wisely seek to help women break their economic dependency upon men; those who provide refuge for women sensibly prohibit men on the premises. But there is a branch of feminist thought which advocates severing all links between women and men for all time. Their core conviction is that any contact with men is harmful. The feminist writer McNay (1991) cautions against this stance: 'Feminist practice should not only be concerned with women ... Feminism can and should encourage change that enhances all members in relationships' (pp. 53–4). Childcare professionals who wish to sever the link do not engage men in childcare work, do not seek to assess the precise role of men in childcare problems which exist, and certainly do not seek to include men in a resolution of the problem. In addition, they have a dismal perception of what their male colleagues may have to offer mothers. Milner's (1993) view that 'men have hijacked the child protection industry' may strengthen these anti-men convictions held by some frontline feminist workers. But the reality is that such convictions are potentially abusive and dangerous to women; they are far removed from the mainstream feminism of writers such as McNay, and Dominelli and McLeod (1989) whose work is dominated by the principle that: 'one person's feelings of self worth should not be built on the denial or denigration of another's. And if women depart from this, they are ceasing to hold true to the spirit and the practice of feminist theory' (p. 82).

Men are undoubtedly often responsible for the abuse of children, or, make a significant contribution to factors leading to mothers abusing their children. Yet, men are often avoided by workers with strong anti-men convictions, leaving mothers isolated and vulnerable in the frontline of intrusive and painful investigations (see Chapters 1 and 8 which describe and explore this matter in detail).

Women and racism

Childcare systems in a multicultural society can be abusive whenever the principles and values upon which they are based derive from a single dominant race and culture. The abuse is more likely if the vast majority of the agencies' personnel belong to that race and culture, and harbour racist attitudes to the differing races and cultures of clients for whom they provide a service. In this section of the chapter, we explore how racism may add to and exacerbate the abuses perpetrated against women by childcare systems.

The integration of racism and the abuse of women We have already noted that the predominent Western culture is steeped in a tradition of patriarchy and sexism. Women are abused on a massive scale within that culture. It is important to emphasize this point, lest one should think that multiculturalism itself has in some way created the problem. Langan (1991b) stresses that race should not be perceived merely as a separate, additional potentially abusive feature; it is in fact another pervasive strand of the oppression of women as a whole: 'it does not simply make the experience of women's subordination greater; it qualitatively changes the nature of that subordination' (1991b: 5). Langan and other feminist writers (Dominelli and McLeod 1989; Day 1992; Milner 1993) concede that feminist therapy and practice for far too long did not incorporate a black perspective, and ignored the accentuated plights of black women clients receiving services from white-dominated social work and childcare agencies. Day highlights the 'white middle class perspective' which 'has rendered black women's lives and the specificity of their experiences invisible' (1992: 17). Langan, however, stresses the imbalance of power between men and women, irrespective of race.

Racist stereotyping Numerous writers have explored the manifestation of racism and its impact upon black people generally. There is, however, little writing on the specific manifestation of racism directed against black mothers. Bryan's (1991) account of work with black single mothers and Currer's (1991) work with Pathan women are notable exceptions. Bryan exposes the myths upon which racist attitudes and practice may be based, for example, that giving birth to illegitimate children 'is the norm for women of Afro-Caribbean origin' or that the young black woman is 'sexually immoral and uninterested in longterm relationships' (1991: 168). There is the myth of the older black woman, 'a matriarch, independent but submissive, a child rearer, God fearing and respectable' (Bryan 1991: 169); and the associated myth noted by Langan (1991b) that the Afro-Caribbean family, with this mythical matriarchal figure at the centre, 'can cope with all the problems of childcare, without external support' (p. 83). The stereotyping of black males may also lead to the abuse of women; they may be perceived as so problematic, that is, aggressive, dangerous, sexually violent etc. (Milner 1993), that they will be avoided even more than men generally are avoided by professionals (see Chapter 8), thus leaving the mother to face professionals alone.

Racism in childcare culture Miles (1991) makes the general point that little attention has been paid to the health beliefs of minority ethnic groups in contemporary Western societies. Currer (1991) however, has made considerable effort to do so with Pathan women, with whom she has worked in Pakistan and Birmingham. Her work is in effect a classic analysis of the inadequacies of the system of healthcare and childcare available to Pathan women, based as it is on narrow, prejudicial perceptions of such issues as: (1) childhood and child development; (2) birth and mothering; (3) social skills; (4) role of medical personnel in the service of mothers; and (5) Ramadan fasting. Regarding social skills (point 3) Currer writes:

> Pathan children's social skills are well developed, yet such skills may not be apparent in (western) child development and educational testing. What they measure may be a very partial view of the child's overall development. This partiality is racist when we give the impression that children of minority groups are less well developed than white children of their own age, or, that their mothers are poor raisers of children. (1991: 45)

Regarding the fourth point, Currer says that Pathan mothers often ignored the advice of health visitors and GPs. They regarded themselves as the experts in infant and childcare, due to their considerable personal, family and community experiences. They would therefore be vulnerable to the undermining of that experience by trained professionals; as Miles (1991) points out, the consequence of the increasing medicalization of childcare has been that health visitors and GPs have imposed their 'expertise' upon mothers, and that 'women's own intuitive knowledge and the accumulated wisdom of the social group become lay, i.e., inexpert, in the eyes of professionals who emphasise that theirs is the only valid and authentic expertise' (p. 201). On the final point, Currer states that the Ramadan fasting by pregnant Pathan mothers is misunderstood by many healthcare and childcare professionals. The practice of fasting has been condemned as dangerous, thus displaying an ignorance of the spiritual importance of the fast, and a lack of trust in the mothers 'underestimating their capacity to act responsibly on the basis of their knowledge of their own health' (1991: 47).

Women and disability

Reference has already been made in this and previous chapters, to the large measure of control imposed upon the lives of women. This attempt to control may constitute abuse. Greater effort to control will be made by government and caring agencies in the case of women experiencing some form of disability. The case of Julie Gates (Channel 4 1994b; Crampton 1994), a blind and deaf single parent mother, highlighted her determination not to be controlled, and also, the extraordinary efforts made by a whole array of childcare professionals striving to enable her to continue caring for her child. No doubt, similar efforts are being made elsewhere by many professionals on behalf of mothers with disabilities. But there are also clear indications of discrimination against them. Distorted perceptions of disability in general, and the mothering capacities of women with disability in particular, can form the core of an additional abusing component in childcare systems. This section briefly looks at this controversial issue, and begins with a well publicized recent case history of a woman with learning difficulties. Booth and Booth's (1994) seminal work on discriminatory practice against parents with learning difficulties, particularly mothers, is a severe indictment of childcare and community care agencies entrusted with the responsibility of empowering them and enhancing their parental and citizen status.

The abuse of women with learning difficulties Childcare agencies have contributed to discrimination against women diagnosed as having learning difficulties or disabilities. The word 'contributed' needs to be stressed, as the abuse of such women has stemmed from a broad base including Parliament, the judiciary, childcare professional organizations, the medical profession, moral philosophers, etc. The most prominent case indicative of this discriminatory trend was that of Jeanette, a 17 year old Sunderland girl with learning difficulties, who in 1987, was, with the approval of the High and Appeal Courts, compulsorily sterilized because she was beginning to exhibit signs of sexual awareness (Wertheimer 1987). Numerous similar cases have followed, with less and less controversy, and it is increasingly likely that sterilization will become automatic in such cases. There are, of course, important questions about parental rights in the case of minors with learning difficulties and other disabilities (Jeanette's parents initiated the process). But numerous ironies are apparent. As Williams (1991) points out, the whole thrust of Care in the Community, and more specifically, the care of people with disabilities, has been in the direction of increasing their autonomy and independence. Williams asks: 'Does it mean that the granting of rights in one area – the right to live in the community and develop relationships – carries with it the denial of right in another area – the right to reproduction and motherhood?' (1991: 155). Women with learning difficulties are perceived as not having the necessary intellectual capacities necessary for motherhood; in fact, emotional wellbeing is more important in child rearing, and there is no evidence or research to indicate that people with learning difficulties are emotionally impaired.

Those who make decisions on whether or not women with disabilities of any kind should be permitted to have children, or be discouraged or prevented from doing so, are nearly always male. The moral argument seems to revolve around the quality of life of the child: society, through its legal and welfare institutions, has assumed the right to prevent conception in the belief that the child is likely to be handicapped in some way. No such moral questions are asked, however, when physically healthy, invariably well-off parents take enormous risks in genetic engineering and *in vitro* fertilization, to have a child for the first time, or, to choose the sex of their child, or, to have a child much later in life; in such cases, damaged foetuses can easily be detected and discarded.

The 'disability' of being a woman In many countries and cultures women are considered to be disabled because of their sex. Girls when born are instantly perceived as a lifelong crippling financial burden. Baby girls are murdered in their thousands, leaving huge imbalances in the male–female population. Often this is open practice, shared by medical and childcare staff and the local population alike. Many doctors in India participate (and enrich themselves) in a flourishing sex diagnosis and abortion industry. Their time is spent not healing the sick, but examining pregnant women to find out if they are going to give birth to a boy or a girl. If the latter, the foetus is likely to be aborted, or the girl murdered when born. The Indian Government deplores the practice and makes strenuous efforts to halt it; but its efforts make little impact upon a practice rooted in a centuries-old tradition, sustained by ceaseless grinding poverty and social convention. In Britain, there have been indications in recent years of doctors and other professionals facilitating the abortion of foetuses of Asian women, for the sole reason that the foetus is that of a girl. This reason may be concealed. An inquest in Leeds (in March 1994) confirmed that an Asian mother who died having an abortion misled Family Planning and medical personnel. The abortion was requested on numerous other grounds; but the real reason why the request was made was because her expected child would be a girl (*Yorkshire Evening Post* 3 March 1994).

Abusive convictions originating in past experiences

So far, we have explored the abuse and potential abuse of women in numerous political, institutional and societal contexts. Such abuses are rampant simply because they stem from attitudes, beliefs and prejudices which are shared by millions of people – professional and lay people alike. The abuses are as common as the sources from which they stem. This next section will explore abuses which may not be quite so common, because their origins lie in very individualistic, private experiences of professional childcare workers. But they are damaging abuses nonetheless.

A manager's problem

Some time ago, a frontline senior practitioner's decision in a child abuse investigation was overruled by her area manager. She had concluded that there were no grounds for removing the child from his single parent mother. The manager insisted that the child be removed and placed in hospital for medical monitoring. The worker later approached the manager to convey her dissatisfaction with his decision. They discussed the case. During this discussion, he repeatedly referred to an experience in his past professional life, in which a child on his caseload had been killed by her mother. He believed he had been negligent in his duty by not monitoring carefully enough. This had made him ultra-cautious ever since. What the worker found so striking about that conversation was the manager's lack of awareness about the nature of the motivation driving him; it was purely emotion and memory-led; the emotions of guilt, fear and anxiety evoked by the memory of his terrible experience. We need to examine this phenomenon, namely, how convictions based upon personal and/or professional experiences (as opposed to mere 'common beliefs') can wittingly and unwittingly lead to the abuse of women in childcare work. Women may be abused as a consequence of either of the following: (1) the workers' professional experience; and (2) the workers' personal experiences (in childhood, adolescence or adulthood), those experiences creating negative perceptions of mothers in vulnerable, oppressive situations.

Past professional experiences

There are many experiences with clients in the past which have the potential for abuse of women in the present, for example, as above if a mother kills a child who is under the supervision of the agency, or, if a mother who has been assessed as trustworthy, breaks that trust by again neglecting her children. Workers are likely to be powerfully affected by these experiences. A sustained cynicism and lack of trust of mothers in general may be the result, a determination never to risk a second chance where children have been abused in the first instance. If that worker has become a manager in childcare, the lack of trust may envelope the frontline staff for whom he or she is responsible: 'they are being too trustworthy as I was ... they are not vigilant enough ... they have not experienced the unreliability of mothers as I have'. 'Professionalism' is incompatible with such potentially abusive subjectivity, but the reality as Sommerfeld and Hughes (1987) established in their research, is that even without such painful past experiences, professionals have a tendency to rely on subjective judgement rather than on professional criteria.

Identification, projection, punishment

Personal experiences in childhood, in family and married life, may also contain the potential for the abuse of women. Black *et al.* (1993) and Russel *et al.* (1993) researched the backgrounds of social workers and other professionals, and discovered an alarmingly high degree of imbalance, dysfunction and mental health problems in the childhoods of the former. How such adverse experiences in childhood manifest themselves in adult professional life is not yet known, but Lawrence's (1992) feminist perspective on the possible impact of the emotional deprivations in the childhoods of female children is, nevertheless, enlightening. She highlights the cultural, structural, and economic contexts which determine the 'subordinate psychology' of women, 'centred on pleasing and affiliation with others rather than on meeting their own needs and asserting their own views' (p. 34). Women's emotional lives have throughout childhood been suppressed. Emotions indicating stress and inability to cope are not tolerated. This is not simply a problem of how women think and feel about the way they are perceived; more realistically, 'women who can't cope are likely to lose their children or their liberty' (p. 37). Lawrence concentrates upon some of the consequences of this 'subordinate psychology' for women entering the caring professions, and asks: if women are 'notoriously bad at taking care of themselves, of meeting their own needs' (p. 45), how can they be effective in fulfilling the needs of clients who are predominently female? 'As copers ourselves, do we unconsciously blame and punish women we see showing that they have difficulties?' (p. 45). Like other researchers (for example, Parton 1990), Lawrence warns of the danger of 'minimizing the real needs of our women clients', perpetuating the patriarchal myth of women as the eternal copers, and, 'reluctant to hear and engage with the depth of their pain and distress' (p. 46). More seriously the professional woman may collude with the client; she may not resist the client's pretence of coping, even when the fact that the client is not coping, is obvious: 'Such unconscious abuse of women clients might include for example, encouraging a severely depressed mother to "carry on" when our professional judgement ought to tell us that she is simply not able to' (p. 46).

Sayers (1991) concentrates upon countertransference as a potentially abusing phenomenon. She identifies abusive countertransference reactions on the part of child protection workers, including that of the young social worker, 'still seeking to become independent of their own families ... wanting to rescue the child to the neglect of the parents' possible strengths and abilities' (p. 89). Sayers emphasizes the differences in countertransference reactions in male and female workers. A male worker who in childhood has helplessly witnessed his mother periodically battered by his father, and who encounters a similar situation in work, may experience powerful feelings of hatred and aggression towards the father. A female worker who recalls an all powerful dominating father and a subordinate mother in her childhood, and who perceives similar characteristics in a current case, may experience powerful feelings of resentment and/or contempt for the mother. Mothers, always more accessible than fathers, will be the main target of these potentially damaging countertransference reactions from a workforce predominantly female. There are occasions when the worker's hostility to mothers (irrespective of whatever type of countertransference is being activated) is so blatant and destructive, that all aspects of professionalism are precluded from the process. Here is one example from an actual case:

> A qualified social worker is given the case of Mary, a 15 year old who is exceedingly unhappy with her mother and stepfather, Mr and Mrs Jones. The parents are seeking social work help because they find Mary unmanageable, and fear that she may be misled by others into giving up school where she has been progressing very well. Over a period of months, the worker records her perceptions of Mrs Jones. Mrs Jones is: 'full of guilt ... extremely aggressive ... has stored up a great deal of resentment against her daughter ... appeared to be very neurotic'. The worker also records similar perceptions of the mother by members of the extended family: an aunt of Mary's thought that Mrs Jones 'needed treatment before she ruined Mary's life'; that she 'was an evil woman who had never been content unless she is hurting someone or blaming someone'. The worker writes of Mary: 'she is a quiet shy girl, who obviously cares for her parents ... she is a placid girl who does not speak up for herself unless really roused ... it seemed to me to be a virtual impossibility that Mary could be aggressive in the home'. The worker suggests a temporary separation, Mary to go to a girls' hostel. A month later, the Officer in Charge gives Mary an ultimatum that if she hasn't stopped lying, drinking, smuggling girls into the hostel late at night and creating mayhem generally, she would have to go. Needless to say, as this file records, the case degenerates into tragedy. Mrs Jones becomes suicidal, Mr Jones becomes more and more threatening to social services whom he holds responsible for his wife's condition, and, Mary helplessly lurches from bouts of alcoholism, to phases of depression and despair. There is no information about the worker's own family history, particularly the relationship with her own mother.

Many childcare professionals who have endured abuse and deprivations in childhood can successfully utilize such experiences to provide the highest quality of service to their clients. Indeed, their motivation to do so and their commitment to vulnerable clients are often greater as a consequence of their experiences. Yet, as Lawrence and Sayers suggest, and as the above case demonstrates, some workers who have endured similar experiences are alternatively motivated. Mothers in particular may suffer enormously as a consequence: they may suffer the impact of a service that is palpably bad; and they may suffer the frustration and self-doubt in not having a clue why a professional person could treat them like that.

Novelty, experiments and experts

This final section explores the abusive potential of a seldom acknowledged feature of childcare agencies, namely, the eagerness of powerfully placed individuals within those agencies to engage in novel, experimental childcare and/or child protection work. At first sight, this may appear a welcome feature, contrasting favourably with many of the well en-trenched abusive features described in this and the following chapter. But it is not as simple as that. Motivation is the crucial factor. One motivation that is always emphasized is that the new approach or method is primarily in the child's best interests; but any scrutiny of what is being done is likely to reveal much more.

Innovation or merely intensifying the abuse?

Childcare agencies are a fertile ground for novel, experimental work, by those who will be quickly perceived as experts in their field. Ostensibly, this work will be directed at children for whom all childcare agencies profess their paramount concern; but the reality is that mothers will be the principal beneficiaries or losers. Sometimes, governments are the initiators of experimental work, responding to a prevailing climate of public opinion and offering unlimited funding to those willing to carry it out. As we have already seen, the current Government's preoccupation with the 'cost' of single parents has led some prominent members to suggest persuading single parents to give up their children for adoption. This would save the Treasury a fortune, and middle class childless couples would be grateful. Another idea being promoted is that which seeks to deny single parents of any state help if they have any more than one child. The model for this experiment lies in New Jersey (and possibly China), perceived by many who have given it neither sufficient time nor scrutiny, as the inevitable and desirable way ahead.

The male 'experts'?

Men are often the driving force behind new directions in childcare and child protection work. Dale *et al.* (1986) developed a potentially abusive model of child protection work criticized by Hooper (1992) for being 'more residual and more pessimistic than the preventative orientation of the 1960s'; Hearn (1990) criticizes the same model, and facetiously refers to Dale and his three male co-authors as 'the male experts' on the problems of mothers in child protection cases. Men are predominantly in the senior and managerial position that enables them to fund, staff, supervise and influence new childcare strategies; they often have more than a professional interest in its perceived success. The most notorious case of the exploitation of a woman by 'expert' 'professional' men, is that of the Californian child known as Genie, locked in her room, tied to the bed, for more than ten years of her childhood (BBC2 1994). Such was the extent of her retardation, that for more than ten years after she was discovered she was the coveted object of every conceivable type of male childcare expert inflicting their own research agendas upon her (so much so, that Genie's mother actually took them to court). The cruel irony was that the experts, whose reputations flowered during their research on Genie, made no progress whatsoever on her plight.

Tens of thousands of murdering mothers?

Another new male expert has recently arrived in the field of child-care (Meadows 1985, 1993a, 1993b; Stephenson 1994). Their subject is Munchausen's syndrome by proxy, in which a parent (invariably a mother) craves attention from professionals and abuses her child (some-times killing the child) to ensure that she gets that attention. Meadows's (1985) article (he is probably the world's leading 'expert' on the subject) is breathtaking in its recommendations; it reads in some places like a black comedy. He stresses the need for the paediatrician in charge of the case to enlist 'the help of a few key members of the staff whom one can rely on to be obsessional' (p. 389) – that is, obsessional in their surveillance of mothers suspected of harming their children. Another strategy is (without her being aware of it): 'searching a mother or her possessions [for articles she may use to harm her child]'; this is a task he may delegate to his subordinates: 'Mothers do leave their locker in their rooms and their bags unattended for brief periods. For a junior doctor to check that there is no drug or poison can be done speedily and without upset' (p. 389). He does add though, that 'I . . . would prefer to do it myself'.

The more recent 'experts' in this field have taken it upon themselves to install hidden cameras in hospital wards, to record what goes on between a suspected mother and her child (Channel 4 1994a; Dobson 1994; Stephenson 1994). The police realize the implications for prosecution and

Figure 5.1 Abusive components and processes in child care systems

	Child care principles misinterpreted, and exploited	Abusive common beliefs	Racism	Discrimination against disability	Abusive convictions arising from past experiences	Novelty experiments, and experts
Politics and politicians						
Hostility to single parents	'The welfare of the child is paramount'	The 'collusive mother'	Abuse of women and racism integrated	The abuse of women with learning difficulties	Child protection governed by fear	Innovations: mothers always available
Moral outrage, new laws, punitive intervention	'No child should be in residential care'	The all-coping 'you'll-manage-it' mother	Racist stereotyping	Perception of 'womanhood' as a disability	Identification	Male experts on women
Remove children		Grandmother knows best	Racism in childcare culture		Protection	Secret videoing of suspected mothers
		Men are not worth bothering about			The need to punish mothers	

have expressed concern (Fox 1994). Thomas (1994) has traced the development of the practice and castigates it for its 'invasion of privacy, for wasting valuable resources' and possibly, for 'deliberately putting children at risk in the interests of catching possible offenders' (p. 967). Mothers do not know when they are suspected, and the criteria for suspecting them has no validity in proper scientific testing or research (Morley 1992). As is to be expected, the male pioneers of these practices are publicizing their 'successes', and, entirely predictably, any question on the morality of the practice provokes the response: 'the child's welfare is paramount'.

We will take the liberty of making another prediction: the practice will spread; many more mothers will be subjected to covert videoing; some mothers' innocent actions will be interpreted as harming their children; they will be apprehended, interrogated, charged and tried, possibly on a wave of public revulsion against such 'crime'; innocent mothers will be found guilty and imprisoned; then later, somewhere, a case will be reopened; a mother will be freed; a public enquiry will be heard, in which the illegality and the immorality of the practice will be exposed. The 'experts' will protest they are the victims of a witchhunt, and the public will revile them because of what they have done to innocent women.

Conclusion

Let us recap now on this first chapter on abusive childcare systems. The potentially abusive components and features which we have addressed are so diverse and numerous that Figure 5.1 may help. In the next chapter we will address the more tangible, less varied, potentially abusive features which exist within the *legal, organizational,* and *procedural* foundations of childcare systems.

6

Abusive childcare systems II

Introduction

This second chapter on abusive childcare systems will concentrate on the three major factors of (1) law and the legal context; (2) organization and structure of childcare agencies; and (3) childcare policies and procedures. These factors differ enormously from those of the previous chapter (though the two are not mutually exclusive); there was a primitive, abstract quality in many of those factors, and their potential for abusing women was not always easily recognized (such as, with certain common beliefs, prevailing political and public climates of opinion; the influence of professionals' past painful experiences upon their present work). No such 'primitiveness' or abstraction exists within the three major foundational pillars which we will now explore; all childcare work is governed by childcare law, the structure and organization of the childcare agency for which one is working, and the childcare policies and procedures which the agency has implemented.

The law

Childcare laws are formulated in the interests of children and their primary carers. They do not always serve those interests. There are numerous reasons for this, some of which have already been referred to. First, the laws may be hastily formulated and enacted as a consequence of public opinion provoked by some tragic event; second, powerful individuals may have launched well supported crusades which pressurize politicians into changing existing laws; third, laws may be interpreted and applied differently to that intended by those who produced them; and fourth, new laws have been formulated on the basis of outdated perceptions of the society in which such new laws must operate. The Children Act 1989 provides numerous examples of the latter; there appears to be no awareness in the Act of the accelerating fragmentation of community and family life, the soaring divorce rate, the fast diminishing number of traditional nuclear families, the dramatic increase in reconstituted families (those fundamental societal changes addressed in the previous chapter). The terminology of the Act – for example, 'rights and responsibilities of the parents . . . rehabilitation to the family . . . natural parents of the child', etc. – conveys the impression (or is it hope) that the traditional nuclear family has remained the lynchpin around which society still revolves. This apparent unawareness of the profound changes in the structure of families and society when childcare laws are being enacted, has implications for how women are treated in childcare work and in court proceedings. Before looking more closely at the Children Act and other legislation, potentially abusive features in the broader legal context and care proceedings in general need to be identified.

The adversarial court

The vast majority of 'parents' who participate in childcare proceedings in court are women; they are either single parent mothers, or, their male partners cannot attend, or choose not to attend. They are key witnesses, to be questioned (if not interrogated) by as many as four solicitors; or even more since the Children Act 1989; Ian Robertson (1993), a solicitor specializing in childcare law writes:

> Children Act cases have become more confrontational. Matters, which would have been straightforward under the old legislation have become obfuscated by the proliferation of parties and their representa- tives, some of whom unfortunately do not sufficiently understand children's law and practice to act in the best interests of the child or their client. (p. 16)

King and Trowell (1992) write about the paradox of using the courts for child welfare. They see the law colonizing childcare through the enactment of more and more childcare laws, yet the nature of law, and its primary goal of simplying the complex, is incompatible with the nature and goals of childcare work. There are no easy solutions in childcare, either in analysis or in resolution. The law's tendency to individualize problems – that is, always to see the cause and sustenance of problems within individual behaviour – precludes the necessary consideration of wider social and economic factors. Thus mothers who have abused their children or have been unable to protect their children may easily be pathologized in the proceedings; and if they manage to protest about their ordeal in court through tears or anger or disgust, the pathology may only be confirmed.

Courts seek speedy and confident expert opinion and assessments. King and Trowell (1992) recall a solicitor on the day of a court hearing requesting a psychiatrist to carry out an on-the-spot assessment of a parent whom the psychiatrist had never met. The Children Act underlines the urgency of assessments (the seven days allowed is woefully inadequate); childcare agencies are cautioned that they may not get the Order they seek if there is, in the opinion of the judge, unnecessary delay (s. 1(2)). But assessments of the quality of care and of the relationships between a parent and a child often require a great deal of time; they require detailed, systematic, recorded observations of parent and child, over long periods. When these are not available, as often they are not, impressions and appearances on the day acquire a significance which they do not warrant. The adversarial nature of the proceedings and the strategic play engaged in by the principal protagonists inhibit mothers either from acknowledging they have abused or have not protected, or, that they are burdened with numerous social, marital, or economic problems contributing to the abuse. This will, of course, label the mother as a parent who refuses 'to admit the existence of problems' which may lead to the additional label that she is beyond any therapeutic help.

King and Trowell (1992) provide a chilling example of the consequences of the adversarial nature of proceedings, and of the court's unrealistic demand for decisive, unambiguous professional expertise. The professional was a child psychiatrist giving evidence in the case of a mother 'with a history of incompetence and neglect'. The psychiatrist was in favour of continuing contact between mother and child, but she believed the child should not return to the mother's care:

> This psychiatrist said that she found herself 'driven into the position of saying 'she's an absolutely appalling mother' and of 'totally annihilating her' by undertaking 'a character assassination' in order to prevent any possibility of the child going home . . . The situation she explained, required her to act strategically in court because she feared that anything said in the mother's favour would be seized upon by the barrister and used as an argument for the child returning home. (1992: 93)

One hopes that the psychiatrist was aware of the consequences of her testimony for the mother's sense of worth, and for the quality of care she could then offer the child during the contacts which the psychiatrist thought so important!

Adoption law

All adoption literature, legislation, policy and procedures use the term 'natural parents', as though professionals are always dealing with the natural father and the natural mother in each adoption case; the reality is that agencies and courts deal predominantly with the natural mothers alone; natural fathers remain as inaccessible or as absent as always; in fact they are now likely to be even more invisible, particularly in adoption work with single parent mothers, as many of them will want to avoid the increasingly discredited Child Support Agency; some may also be under threat from the families of the women they have made pregnant.

The birth mother has always been considered and treated in adoption law as the least important of the three parties, that is, the child, prospective adopters and the child's mother. Goodacre's (1966) well known research study *Adoption Policy and Practice*, which was highly influential in adoption law which followed, did not even include the natural mothers among the respondents. Lowe's (1993) research on the use of freeing orders was carried out without any contact with mothers, despite the fact that mothers are principally affected by freeing orders. (Lowe and colleagues acknowledge this fact and are currently engaged in new research which will embrace the views and feelings of mothers.) In the case of reconstituted families and older children, adoption law is blatantly discriminatory; when a stepfather wishes to adopt the children of a family he has joined, the mother of the children (who has likely been caring for her children since birth) must surrender her parental status for the duration of the application, and become, just like her new partner, a prospective adoptor. Phillips's (1993) research on step-parent adoptions gives some indication of how offensive this process is to the mothers involved.

The Government's White Paper proposing new legislation on adoption (DoH 1993) does nothing to alter the lowly position held by mothers in the adoption triangle; indeed, it is obvious that the *raison d'être* for the proposals is to improve the experiences of the prospective adoptive parents, who, as Rickford (1993) points out, have the 'the highest media profile and strongest political clout of the parties involved in the adoption triangle' (p. 19). The white paper is in fact another classic example of politicians being pressurized by media and public to introduce legislation which will in effect be more abusive of mothers than existing legislation. (Some of the pressure on this occasion arose from a highly publicized adoption case in Norfolk, in which an Anglo-Asian couple were refused permission to adopt a mixed race child (*Community Care* 11 April 1993). The media generally believed the couple were badly treated, but the adoption panel's decision was vindicated by subsequent enquiry.)

Freeing orders

The Houghton (1972) report was responsible for the introduction of freeing orders, which came into effect with the 1976 Adoption Act (s. 18). The intention was to minimize the uncertainty and indecision which characterized the period between a mother giving initial consent and the court granting (or refusing) an adoption order (Terry 1976). A freeing order vests the parental rights and duties relating to the child in the adoption agency; it extinguishes the natural parents' or guardians' parental rights and duties. Its effect overall is: 'as if the order were an adoption order and the agency were the adopters' (Pearce 1984: 17). In the light of this powerful order, Houghton's vision of consensus between natural parent and adoption agency, enabling them to make joint application for a freeing order, has proven naively idealistic (Lambert *et al.* 1989; Lowe 1993). Howe *et al.* (1992) are critical about the effect of the orders:

Mothers who fight this nightmarish decision (i.e., the agency applying for a freeing order) and lose, not only experience all the pain felt by mothers who voluntarily relinguish their baby, they suffer the added horror of having their children forcibly removed and adopted against their wishes. (p. 5)

Contrary to what Houghton believed, applications for freeing orders have led to a dramatic increase in the number of contested adoptions (Lambert *et al.* 1989; Lowe 1993). Generally, mothers who willingly place their child for adoption endure trauma and distress, and long-term psychological difficulties (Winkler and Van Keppel 1984); but those increasing number of mothers who actually lose (and most of them will lose) their children after protracted conflicts with adoption agencies, fought out in the glare of court proceedings, will suffer even more. Triseliotis (1993) remarks that 'the prospect of introducing into adoption the adversarial procedure that have marred divorce proceedings and access issues ... is horrifying' (p. 3); this is precisely what appears to be happening, according to Lowe (1993).

Adopted child's right to trace birth parent

The 1975 Children Act gave adults who had been adopted in childhood the right to see their birth records (s. 26). This in effect enables them to trace and make contact with their natural parents. Many mothers would of course wish for this to happen, but no agency has accepted responsibility for preparing mothers for the challenge which such encounters pose. Proposed changes in adoption law (DoH 1993) will increase the adopted child's right to access to information about their birth parents, again with no corresponding commitment to helping the parent(s) cope with the consequences. Howe *et al.* (1992) have recorded many of the fears and apprehensions shared by a group of birth mothers in response to these increasing rights granted to their children (see Chapter 7).

The Children Act 1989

The Children Act 1989 gives little indication that those who formulated it were aware of the fact that childcare agencies predominantly work with one parent families; the notion that the two parent, nuclear family is as prevalent and permanent as it has always been, pervades much of the Act. An underlying theme, vigorously promoted throughout, is of both natural parents exercising rights and responsibilities in respect of their children. This may appear reasonable and commonsensical, if both parents have equal power, influence, independence, security, accommodation, financial means, job security and commitment to the child. This is unlikely to be the case. To encourage, even worse, to demand that a father exercises his parental duties and responsibilities in respect of children to whom he may not be genuinely committed, a child cared for by a mother lacking confidence, power and assertiveness, is fraught with risk to both mother and child. In a childcare legal world primarily adversarial (and made more so by the Act), reality and truth can easily be sacrificed at both the child's and mother's expense.

The Act permits greater surveillance of parents (Cooper 1993), but this will in effect mean mothers in inner city areas becoming the main target of tighter control and surveillance (Parton 1990; Hooper 1992). Langan (1991b), Cooper (1993) and Robertson (1993) draw attention to the cost saving and contradictory features in the Act: while recognizing that 'services to families' are the first step in the prevention of abuse, there is no concrete financial commitment ensuring that such services can be provided: 'The Act reflects both the state's attempts to regulate family life and its desire to reduce the public contribution to childcare' (Langan 1991b: 78). It is single mothers, already the predominant carers of children, who need that contribution raised. Langan also highlights possible consequences of the abolition of 'voluntary care'; this was a commonly used catch-all provision of the 1948 Children's Act which obscured the distinction 'between children needing day care as a welfare provision and those whom the courts decide require council care as a protective or coercive measure' (p. 80). Langan believes that private childcare will flourish, while the 'most disadvantaged children will be "selectively" accommodated in a residual, stigmatized, and under-resourced public sector' (p. 80).

Some initially regarded the Act as an abusive parents' charter. Childcare professionals now have to be much more rigorous and systematic in their assessments and recommendations; a much more comprehensive report and proven good quality alternative care is needed if the recommendation is to remove a child. But the reality is that Local Authorities are still left with enormous discretion and little need for professional or ethical criteria in certain sections of the Act.

The Act implicitly encourages *partnership with parents*. The concept of partnership has been very prominent in childcare literature in recent years, chiefly because of the emphasis given to it in the Department of Health's (1991b) *Working Together*. This emphasis was made because of the exposure, of parents being marginalized, and/or ignored in many child abuse enquiry reports, particularly Cleveland (Butler-Sloss 1988). The Act does not define partnership, consequently, childcare agencies have defined it and implemented it in whatever way they saw fit. There is enormous variation in this implementation, ranging from the commitment to achieve partnership and make it work, to token gestures without substance. The Act's heavy and pervasive emphasis upon the 'welfare of the child', a principle on which it is absolutely clear, and its lack of clarity and direction on the principle of partnership, has led many practitioners and managers to see the two principles as incompatible. Partnership implies equality, but parents (O'Hagan 1994b), practitioners (Newman 1993) and researchers (Daines *et al.* 1990) have all voiced scepticism about the quality of partnership that may be achieved. The most visible manifestation of the goal of partnership is the policy of parental participation in child protection work; but lone single parents (male and female) realize that 'partnership', in the context of all-embracing procedures for child protection work, is mere rhetoric. The concept of partnership and how it is applied in child protection work will be explored in more detail in Chapter 8.

Child Support Agency (CSA)

This agency was established by law in 1988. Its principal aim was to ensure that absent fathers contributed to the maintenance of their children. The Agency has fast become an unmitigated disaster, for mothers, fathers and children alike. Reputable pressure groups have been inundated by cases of harassment by CSA officers, interrogation of mothers about the where-abouts of fathers, demands made of fathers for astronomical payments which cannot possibly be met. Middle class fathers with secure well paid jobs are particularly vulnerable; despair and suicides have been recorded; men have given up working because CSA demands on their salary simply make it more economical not to work; no less than 18 different pressure groups have been formed, affiliated to the national 'Network Against The Child Support Agency'; these opposition pressure groups are supported by virtually every national and local newspaper. The Government actually conceded to some of their criticisms and made changes; but many of the groups have made it clear that they seek nothing less than the abolition of the CSA (BBC2 1994b).

How then, can the Child Support Agency be perceived as oppressive to women, when the media have persistently presented examples of the suffering which it has inflicted upon men? Therein lies part of the answer: men, particularly middle class professional men, knowledgeable and confident, have had no great difficulty in organizing and mobilizing against the CSA (and already having achieved some amendments). But uneducated, inarticulate, unconfident poverty stricken young mothers, are not so lucky. It is these mothers who stand in the way of the ultimate prize for the CSA, namely, money (everyone now realizes that the CSA is merely an extension of the Treasury; its original governing principle to ensure that parents fulfilled their obligations to provide for their children has been lost in the effort to reduce state expenditure. Figures which can demonstrate this reduction, and commissions for those most effective in achieving it, are the principal motivating factors). Women who refuse to cooperate with the agency, who refuse to divulge the whereabouts of the father, who refuse to answer questions of intimacy about their relationship with the father (for example, questions about sexual intercourse, the use of contraception, denial of paternity, artificial insemination, etc., as disclosed by the 'Blue books' of CSA, leaked to the *Mail on Sunday* 16 January 1994), are in for a very rough ride indeed, including the possibility of reduction in their state benefits. This questioning itself is an abuse, and many young mothers will give in to the subtle and not-too-subtle ways of their professional interrogators. Therein lies the remaining part of the answer: CSA officers will no longer be around to witness the consequences of their actions such as the possible feelings of revulsion in revealing matters of great intimacy or the fear of the partner whose whereabouts mothers have been pressurized to disclose. And who else may some fathers made poor by astronomical increases in maintainence payments vent their wrath upon, with impunity? Certainly not the anonymous bureaucrats who eventually catch up with them. As one father victim commented (*Independent on Sunday* 19 September 1993), relationships are fragile and fraught enough without this additional deeply divisive agency.

Abusive structures and organization

The structure and organization of childcare agencies can impact favourably or adversely upon the quality of services they provide. Quality of service in organizations generally can be determined by: (1) leadership; (2) the degree of stability or change within the agency; (3) the motivation for change; (4) supervision; (5) the extent of local political influence to which agencies may be subject; (6) the flexibility of systems within the agency;

and (7) the degree of independence and autonomy which may be exercised by frontline staff. Each of these factors will now be explored for their significance to the quality of service mothers receive.

Leadership

Four male Directors of British social services departments – namely, Cleveland, Rochdale, the Orkneys and Nottingham, were criticized in recent child protection enquiry reports. Three were compelled to resign; another moved elsewhere. All four were criticized not for abusing power, but, on the contrary, for a poor quality of management and leadership in particular cases and events. Two of the reports identified subordinates who had exercised significant influence on the course of events. Many of their actions and strategies remain as inexplicable (in terms of professional and ethical standards) as had their leaders' failure to be able to predict the ultimate result. The lack of strong, intelligent leadership will eventually manifest itself in the quality of childcare work offered at various levels in the department; if such leadership continues, frontline work can deteriorate from minor deviations (for example, ignoring certain principles or procedures), to the most blatant abuse of clients. In childcare, many of those clients will be disempowered single mothers, least able to resist such abuse.

Stability or change

Agencies subjected to persistent change in management, structure and personnel, cannot provide a reliable, professional and effective service. Agencies which are stable, have minimal change, and whose policies are underpinned by an enduring, well tested philosophy and practice, are far more likely to provide such a service. Mothers are the principal clients of childcare agencies, contacted and seen even more often than the children themselves. Many of these mothers have been the victims of imper-manency, unreliability, betrayal, chaos and confusion, in both their childhoods and married lives. The agencies to which they may turn for rescue, or which may impose themselves statutorily in the interests of the children, often demonstrate that they are nothing more than a mirror image of that impermanency, unreliability, betrayal, chaos and confusion. This may sound severe criticism; it is nothing more or less than provable fact, to be substantiated by any frontline workers who have worked with childcare agencies for a reasonable period since 1970. Virtually every child abuse enquiry report (for example, DHSS 1974; Blom-Cooper 1985; Butler-Sloss 1988; Levy and Kahan 1991; NCB 1993) has identified these characteristics, brought about in the main by ceaseless change (and occasionally by industrial action), as significant factors in the deterioration of quality of services to the families in question. Mothers, as the primary carers in frequent contact with agency personnel (indeed, often the only adult family member in contact with the agencies), bear the brunt of this deterioration.

Motivation

The motivation for changes in the structure and organization of childcare agencies may stem from: new government policy or guidelines; the conclusions and recommendations of enquiry reports; cost-cutting; or the appointment of a new director for the agency. There is no known major structural or organizational change within any childcare agency motivated by the specific purpose of improving the service offered to mothers, or to lessen the risk of abusing women. Motivations underpinning the changes usually stem from much broader aims, such as providing a better service for the community as a whole (at least, that is the laudable motivation given for staff and public consumption). But the ceaselessness remains constant! That is to say that no sooner are major changes in childcare agencies completed than someone significant enough (usually a newly appointed director) finds it necessary to make further changes. This demonstrates either a naive conviction about the efficacy of change itself, or a deception as to the real motivation for change. On one point we can be certain: mothers and children on the receiving end of the chaos, impermanency and unreliability which invariably result from major change in childcare agencies, are never informed or asked for their opinions before such change takes place. Thus countless mothers are suddenly told, for example, that their health visitor has resigned, been promoted or moved; their social worker is now temporarily acting as team leader and unable to see his clients – but a replacement is urgently being sought; their community midwife has been transferred; well established services (for example, the drop-in centre; the child sexual abuse team; the welfare rights section) have been wound up; that the responsibilities of everyone are being redefined and dramatically changed, etc. Mothers may be excused a little scepticism on hearing that these changes have all been motivated in *their* interests!

Supervision

One of the most common casualties of change within childcare systems is supervision. Good quality supervision necessitates commitment, preparation, dedication, regularity and dependability (precisely the qualities sacrificed by ceaseless change). The lack of good quality supervision has been highlighted in every single child abuse enquiry report. Moore (1988) is scathing in her criticism of systems which do not offer quality supervision. Many frontline workers feel abandoned or betrayed by those responsible for supervising them. Mothers may feel precisely the same about the frontline workers, who often flounder on, in a sea of administrative and organizational chaos surrounding them, overloaded, unsupported, burnt-out. Little wonder then that mothers lose faith in the system, and, as many of the enquiry reports reveal, become more enmeshed in and dependent upon men who pose major threats to the child. This is not an argument in favour of a dependency culture; it is merely an acknowledgement that much of childcare and child protection work is complex and is often crisis oriented (particularly in the initial stage). The very least mothers deserve is that workers can be relied upon, and that they (the workers) have not become cynical, disillusioned and burnt-out as a consequence of the poor quality of supervision they receive. 'Burn-out is lethal' says Moore (1988); 'Caring staff start to make stereotyped responses and become afraid of change' (p. 26).

Implications for quality of care

Childcare agencies and the training establishments which provide qualified staff for them, consistently emphasize the importance of permanency and reliability in the relationship between the child and his/her primary carer. There is ample research evidence to justify this emphasis (Crittenden and Ainsworth 1989; Crittenden 1990; Aldgate 1991). It is a curious fact that childcare managers and trainers seldom emphasize the importance of the permanency and reliability of services offered by childcare agencies. Seldom does the agency manager/supervisor reveal any awareness that this goal of permanency and reliability between primary carer and child, sought after so persistently by staff, is greatly facilitated by agencies and staff who are perceived by mother and child to be permanent and reliable.

Political influence

Politicians, local and national, can influence the quality of services to specific groups of clients. We have recently witnessed how very prominent politicians generated a blatantly anti-single mother campaign. We have also seen how politicians joined and enthused about the anti-child sexual abuse crusade in 1986–8 (until of course, things went disastrously wrong, and they then quickly turned on the crusade itself). Childcare agencies may be influenced by their local political masters in various ways, which may worsen the plight of mothers and children: for example, local councillors may decide to close precious facilities such as family centres, or residential homes offering respite care for mothers of disabled children or children with learning difficulties. There may be a powerful core group of ideologues in the committees responsible for childcare agencies – religious

fundamentalists, extreme feminists, male chauvinists, fanatical mone-
tarists – any one of whom can exert pressure upon the management of
agencies, leading to oppressive and/or abusive practices at the frontline. It
is not improbable that the Government's recent anti-single parent
campaign was welcomed by some local authority social services committees.

Probably the two most serious examples of alleged political influence
detrimental to childcare services are those of Orkney (Black 1992) and
Westminster. Prior to February 1991, when nine children were removed,
some forcibly, from their homes in Orkney, it is alleged that The Orkney
Islands Council increasingly exercised influence over the once highly
regarded Children's Panel system which operated throughout Scotland. A
long serving member of the Panel, Mrs Laughton, resigned at the same
time, making public her concern that the Panel had been fast losing its
independence. There is little doubt in the report by Lord Clyde (1993) and
Black (1992) that political influence contributed to the genesis and
developments leading to the events of February 1991. Westminster
Council was the subject of a different kind of report (District Auditor's
report, *The Times* 7 January 1994; BBC1 1994). Councillors allegedly kept
homes vacant while various groups, one of the largest being that of single
mothers and their children, remained homeless. The properties were
eventually sold to better-off Conservative voters.

Inflexibility of childcare systems

Childcare agency systems have been criticized (see for example, Butler-
Sloss 1988) for being uncertain about their role and responsibilities. In
attempting to counter these criticisms, and to be more effective in the
service of children, management have often insisted on watertight
structures and processes for all phases of involvement in particular cases.
Despite the high degree of instability and change in childcare agencies
(already referred to in this chapter), they can still somehow manage to
maintain these inflexible processes. Howitt (1992) researched numerous
cases of parents wrongly suspected of abuse and identified a process he
termed 'ratcheting'. He claims that childcare agencies have firmly established channels upon which they move in one direction only. It is
extremely difficult for them to reverse, even if the situation warrants it. For
example, an investigation leading to a case conference is not likely to be
reversed by late information exonerating parents from any responsibility
for abuse.

There are numerous examples of 'ratcheting' in the enquiry reports
dealing with child sexual abuse cases (Butler-Sloss 1988; Justice Brown
1991; Clyde 1993). Howitt gives the example of children being taken into
care: numerous factors may have led to this decision such as absent

parents, neglect, inadequate caring, or, the presence of someone who has consistently abused the child. Yet even if these factors are removed, it does not automatically lead to the child being returned. Further investigation may be carried out, new conditions set, a tight hold of the case maintained – all this is indicative of the inflexibility of the system and the difficulty the agency may have in 'letting go'. The agency will of course rightly argue the necessity of vigilance, the paramountcy of ensuring protection by minimizing risk; but this kind of inflexibility itself can generate an anxiety and distrust which may actually increase risk. Many single parent mothers will be more vulnerable to these seemingly irreversible processes, and least likely to be able to resist them. They can be, in effect, the antithesis of agency support which is vital to mothers, and they can seriously reduce the level of self-confidence and hope upon which any rehabilitation must be based.

Rehabilitation will depend much upon assessment. Family centres make a major contribution to comprehensive assessment. There are many excellent family centres flexible enough to embrace all the challenges and opportunities which mothers and their children may bring, with staff determined to respond to all aspects of mothers' predicaments, including economic and environmental aspects. But there are others much less flexible, justifying Statham's (1987) perception of right-wing ideological motivation in the growth of family centres. This is borne out to some extent by Holman's (1988) study, which revealed some negative perceptions of mothers by family centre staff who pursued a deliberate policy of excluding mothers; consequently mothers feel even more disempowered, more inadequate, thus vindicating the initial assessment which has caused intervention by the 'system' in the first instance.

Lack of independence and autonomy of frontline staff

Frontline staff will realize quicker than most how inflexible structures and systems can be grossly unfair to vulnerable client groups, and that they themselves are often as helpless as the vulnerable in attempting any kind of deviation interpreted as risk-taking. Milner (1993) writes of the additional tiers of inspection which child protection agencies are for ever introducing (usually following on some child abuse tragedy); these demand that 'deadlines are met', are quick to criticize, yet offer 'no positive support or praise' (p. 57).

Whereas management has constructed systems and processes which generally play safe with all cases, and which do not differentiate between the nuclear family and single mothers, frontline childcare workers have no such 'luxury'; they are acutely aware of the overwhelming prevalence of single parent mothers; of the way inflexible systems and irreversible processes can cause distress and despair to them, and of the adverse impact this has on the quality of care they provide for their children. Milner (1993) likens the social worker to a ballet mistress, 'urging the prima ballerina [that is, the mother] even on to further effort without any support from management' (p. 60). Frontline workers may have a dilemma in this realization. They may find it difficult to conceal from the mother their conviction that it is the system that is at fault. O'Hagan (1994) revealed a significant number of cases in which this dilemma arose. 'I know it's not the social worker's fault' was a common utterance among parents. Alleviating their disquiet or guilt by revealing it to the mother is of no service at all to the latter; on the contrary, it is likely to convince her that the 'system' is indeed cruel. When structures and processes within childcare agencies stifle the creativity of frontline staff, compel them to concentrate on the negative aspects of the mother's predicament, reduce them to mere mechanical functionaries of a system driven by fear of mistakes made in the past, then the quality of childcare service offered to parents and children will be minimal, and the potential for abuse of single mothers in particular, unlimited.

Policies and procedures

Childcare policies and procedures are formulated with reference to law, expert and/or public opinion, and research findings. None of these reference points guarantee that policy and procedures will prevent the abuse of women or guarantee the protection of the child. For example, Ferguson (1993) writes about an infamous child sexual abuse case in which a mother in frequent contact with workers over many years, endured severe battering throughout those same years, at the same time as her daughter was enduring sustained sexual abuse by the same man (that is, the husband/father). Ferguson states that the childcare workers acted 'in the context of [existing] laws, procedures, and available resources' (1993: 4). The reference point in Cleveland (Butler-Sloss 1988) was so-called expert opinion (O'Hagan, 1990). The Director was advised by these 'experts' to adopt a procedure whereby if sexual abuse were diagnosed in a medical examination, then a Place of Safety Order should be sought and the child removed. Procedures were also found inadequate in the case of Kimberly Carlile (Greenwich 1987), particularly in respect of anonymous referrals. Sone (1993) describes a women's support group set up based on the conviction that the investigative process by child protection workers would always remain a traumatic experience for mothers, irrespective of whatever procedures are in operation. Malcolm and O'Hagan's (1994) research reveals wide discrepancies in the implementation of policy and procedures on parental participation. King and

Trowell (1992) write of the 'tendency for policy to be ideologically driven rather than determined by the needs of individual children' (p. 29).

Abusive policies and procedures may stem from – and help to sustain – some of the abusive organizational and structural features of agencies explored in the previous section. Many childcare agencies still operate on the basis of potentially abusive child protection policies. For example, policies which emphasize differences, or, even worse, conflict between the needs of the child and the needs of the primary carer, and which repeatedly stress that the child's needs are paramount, can very easily blind workers to the reality that there are profound mutual needs between primary carer and child, and/or that the greatest potential for fulfilling the needs of the child usually lies within the capacity of the primary carer, more so than the child's removal to residential or foster home. More specifically, policies and procedures are almost certain to lead to the abuse of women when they: (1) do not discriminate between non-abusing mothers and the abuser; (2) ignore violence perpetrated against women; (3) do not recognize the particular vulnerability of single parent mothers to the anonymous referrals alleging that they are abusing their children; (4) encourage workers to concentrate upon mothers and ignore men; (5) are contradictory in their instructions to workers (for example, encouraging workers to establish trust and compelling workers to break that trust); (6) facilitate excuse making for bad practice; and (7) permanently label mothers.

Non-abusing mothers

When someone makes a referral alleging that a child has been non-accidentally injured, an elaborate process involving administrators and professionals is set in motion long before the precise cause and context of the injury has been established. The identity of the perpetrator is a crucial issue; it may not be the primary carer; it may have been the father, an uncle, a sibling, a neighbour, a grandparent; but, nevertheless, policy and procedures set in motion a process in which the mother of the child is likely to be investigated, and may have to tolerate medical examinations, case conferences and court proceedings. Additionally, she may be subjected to the emotional blackmail associated with the policy of getting the alleged abuser removed. Many procedures simply fail to discriminate between the non-abusing mother and the abuser. This lack of discrimination and its consequential trauma is a consistant theme in Hooper's (1992) aptly named book *Mothers Surviving Child Sexual Abuse*. Workers may sometimes attempt to discriminate by being as supportive and helpful to the mother as they possibly can, but they will be procedure-bound to maintain the mother of the child at the centre of the investigation and everything that proceeds from it, and they will be compelled to enforce procedure whether the mother likes it or not (for example, ensuring the child is medically examined, convening a case conference, etc.). There are many occasions when workers are convinced (on sound professional and ethical grounds) that there is no need for all the elaborate, intrusive, paraphernalia of procedural responses and actions; but procedures must be adhered to nevertheless. Chapter 8 contains details of one such case, conveying the nature and extent of the abuses too frequently incurred through procedures.

Ignoring domestic violence against women

Childcare policies and procedures invariably focus upon women as the principal primary carer; but they seldom encourage or enable workers to help women regularly subjected to domestic violence. There are four common abuses of battered women in childcare work. These abuses are directly attributable to policy and procedure, or, they are a likely consequence.

The first is that policy and procedure do not address the problem: if, as is usual, there is no mention of domestic violence in policy and procedure, it is hardly likely that workers will feel confident in tackling it, nor any compulsion to record it. Thus the workers at the family centre in the case of Toni Dales (NCB 1993) did not record Toni's mother's black eye, because they 'did not know what to do about domestic violence beyond listening and giving some support' (p. 13). The authors recall numerous instances of domestic violence referrals being investigated, and workers concluding that there was no need for social services to be involved because only the mother was getting hit! Hegarty (1993) puts it bluntly: 'How can you promote the welfare of children, if you do not protect their mothers' (p. 9).

The second abuse is that battered women are stereotyped: Ross and Glisson (1991) provide research evidence of much stereotyping in which battered women are perceived as masochistic, insulting, provocative, masculine, domineering, etc. They claim that 'social workers are likely to target their interventions at these stereotyped characteristics, rather than focussing on the abuser' (p. 82).

The third abuse is that battered women's predicament is redefined: women often refer themselves to professionals because the battering is intolerable; professionals often respond by redefining the mother's experience of violence into a criticism of the quality of care she provides for her children (McWilliams and McKiernan 1993; Milner 1993).

Fourth, the feelings and actions of battered women are misinterpreted: fear and terror are common feelings among women persistently battered; such feelings (and the attempts to conceal them) may dictate reponses which workers misinterpret as guilt, lack of cooperation, or hostility. These

misinterpretations will have serious consequences for relationships between mother and agency.

Anonymous referrals

Anonymous referrals are a source of anxiety to both parents and
workers. Single parent mothers are particularly vulnerable to anonymous referrals from estranged, vindictive partners, critical neighbours,
or even concerned professionals. Child protection policies and procedures usually say very little about anonymous referrals, and they
never give any indication that those formulating them are aware of the
risks and complexity of the task of responding to such referrals. 'A
referral is a referral and all referrals should be treated the same' seems to
be the general idea in policy. Referral taking generally has never been
regarded as seriously as it should in childcare work (O'Hagan 1989,
1993); consequently, it is often done inadequately. Thorpe's (1994)
research on referrals reveals that 70 per cent of them did not lead to
intervention, and that an alarmingly high percentage of referrals were
allegations of neglect against single parents.

Anonymous referrals are particularly difficult for workers; the referrer
often projects their own anxiety onto the worker, who may then fail to
scrutinize the available information, or who may be inhibited from asking
crucial questions (the answers to which could rapidly expose the authen-
ticity or otherwise of the referral). The authors recall a case in which a
single parent mother was the subject of no less than six unsubstantiated
anonymous referrals alleging abuses of various kinds over a ten month
period; the fact that so many unsubstantiated allegations had been made in
the past, and that each one had necessitated a deeply offensive visit and
investigation, made no impact on the quality of the referral that followed.
The implication here is that even before a childcare agency begins an
investigation on a referral about a single parent mother and her child(ren),
there is a strong possibility that the contact and referral making itself
already constitute an abuse. Policy and procedure contribute to the
inadequacy of referral taking through a lack of specific guidelines and
instructions to frontline staff. Inadequate referrals can often lead to
inadequate investigations in which unsupported single mothers are the
main victims. Some childcare agencies have policies which permit
childcare professionals (for example, health visitor, GP, teacher, etc.) to
make anonymous referrals. Their anonymity is protected. This is a gross
abuse of professional privilege, contrary to numerous principles about
honesty and integrity in the relationship between client and worker.
Chapter 8 explores the abusive potential in referral taking with the help of
an actual case, and Chapter 11 suggests necessary changes in policy and
procedure on referrals.

Focusing on women, ignoring men

Policy and procedure facilitate a potentially abusive habit which will be exposed throughout this text – namely, concentrating on the mother of the child and ignoring male partners who may be significant in the childcare/ child-abuse situation. This concentrating upon women and ignoring men occurs throughout all phases of childcare work. Referral forms, forms to be used in investigation, assessment, case conferences, court reports, reviews, etc., all provide ample space for information on the parent(s) of the child; but this is nearly always the mother. Very few forms have specific sections for male partners who may or may not be the natural parent of the child. Milner (1993) draws attention to the Department of Health's widely used guidelines on comprehensive assessment (DoH 1988), in which most of the questions can only be addressed to the mother. Policy and procedure never caution workers about the need to explore the influence of male partners, their background, family history, personality, etc., which are all factors to be thoroughly explored in profiling the mother.

The child abuse enquiry reports provide many examples of this tendency. The father of Sukina (Bridge 1991), was severely ill-treated as a child, but this information emerged only after he had beaten her to death. Discussions in case conferences and case conference reports are particularly prone to this imbalance; they are likely to be dominated by information about the woman; the man may even escape mere mention. There are numerous causes for this concentration upon mothers and the neglect/avoidance of their partners. A primary cause is that the policies and procedures often stem from research which has precisely the same imbalance. Childcare and adolescent research is overwhelmingly preoccupied with mothers (Phares 1992). The amount of research which has considered the influence of fathers is minuscule in comparison. Pilgrim and Rogers (1993) make the same point about research in mental health; it invariably concentrates upon women. They suggest that such concentration by researchers is part of the problem: 'in attempting to make women more visible, some feminist scholars may have made men relatively invisible' (p. 43). This may equally apply in the field of childcare. The over-concentration on mothers and the ignoring or avoidance of men is the most prominent characteristic of abusive childcare systems. It is an issue of such importance that it warrants a chapter of its own (see Chapter 9).

Ousting men, blackmailing women

There is, however, one emerging policy which does not ignore men; it is called 'ousting' (PAIN 1990b; Howitt 1992). The objective is to remove men from homes in which, it is alleged, they have sexually abused children, or, in which it is believed they pose a threat of doing so. The police are sometimes relied upon to implement this policy. Childcare workers need have no contact with the men; they can effectively implement the policy by what they do and say to the mothers of the children concerned. Removing the alleged or suspected perpetrator is generally regarded as superior to the alternative action of moving a child. The principles underpinning this policy are now enshrined in the Children Act which compels local authorities to pay or provide for alternative accommodation for alleged abusers. It has taken some time for professionals to discover how complex and dangerous the ousting strategy is, and, how unprincipled it can be. More specifically, it is a strategy often dependent upon the emotional blackmail of the mother of the child, that is: 'if he doesn't go, your child will be removed'. Parents Against Injustice (PAIN) produced a paper in 1990 on ousting, setting out the legal, moral and practice issues involved (PAIN 1990b). Hooper (1992) provides case histories in which the ousting concept is carried to extremes. There are many examples of 'ousting' and the consequential emotional blackmailing of mothers in the authors' own experiences (O'Hagan 1989). The practice will be explored in more detail in Chapter 11.

Contradictions

Policy and procedure make contradictory demands upon childcare workers (Hooper 1992). For example, they stress the importance of gaining the trust of parents and demand that that trust may be breached in the interests of the welfare of the child. Gaining trust is relatively easy when the parent is a young single mother. When the mother then confides in the worker, the worker is duty bound to report any information pertinent to the welfare of the child. The mother may then feel betrayed by the worker. This is an inescapable dilemma for the worker, yet few workers go out of their way on first contact to let parents know of this paramount duty to inform other agencies, including the police, of any relevant information the parents may reveal. Nor does policy encourage them to reflect upon the contradiction inherent here. Policy emphasizes the importance of marital harmony and stability, yet may demand that workers take action which fragments the family unit, such as by removing children, or compelling an alleged abuser to leave the home. Policy stresses and demands child protection, but compels workers to act in ways which are demonstrably abusive towards children, such as removing children from physical and sexual abuse, and subjecting them to unplanned inadequate alternative care certain to cause emotional and psychological abuse. Policy aims to empower mothers and enhance their self-esteem, yet it encourages workers to register children 'at risk' and/or to label mothers 'inadequate', or some other derogatory term, as the only means of gaining necessary resources (Hooper 1992; Milner 1993).

Facilitating excuse-making for bad practice

Policies and procedures are often a lifeline for childcare workers whose actions provoke the wrath of their clients: 'it is the department's policy ... I had no choice in the matter ... I had to stick to procedures', etc. Such utterances may rescue them from unpleasant and potentially violent confrontations. Senior managers will also exploit the potential of policy and procedure for excuse making: a Director of social services said that 'he was satisfied that social workers had followed correct procedures' after the death of Sudio Rouse (*The Observer* 1991). Similar remarks were made in many other child abuse tragedies, and particularly during the exposure of events in Cleveland; workers were said to be only 'carrying out policy ... strictly adhering to procedures', etc. When these utterances are merely an excuse for bad practice they intensify the mothers' sense of helplessness and despair, silence them, and strengthen their conviction about the injustices of 'the system'.

Conclusion

It has been necessary to devote two chapters to a concept increasingly used by both parents and critics of childcare practice, namely: 'abusive childcare systems'. It is a convenient turn-of-phrase, giving the impression of a sinister, pervasive, all-embracing, system, in which the component parts (or subsystems) are related. And each of the components is constructed or formed to play a part in the system's primary goals, that is, consolidating and increasing its malign power and influence over parents and their children; protecting and defending itself from any kind of external scrutiny; and abusing parents who are an obstacle to the system achieving those goals. This impression had to be exposed for the fiction that it is: **There is no grand conspiratorial system in the world of childcare.**

Yet childcare abusive systems do exist and women are the principal victims. These two chapters have explored the many and diverse factors causing or contributing to such abuse, directly or indirectly, wittingly or unwittingly. Chapter 5 began by identifying the component parts of abusive systems, particular childcare professional groups most likely to abuse, and possible motivations underpinning the abuses. It then explored the less obvious, more primitive contributory factors in abusive childcare systems; these were: (1) the prevailing political climate and political opportunism within that climate; (2) the perversion of childcare principles; (3) abusive common beliefs; (4) racism; (5) distorted perceptions of disabled women; (6) potentially abusive convictions arising from past experiences; and (7) novelty, experimentation, and 'expertise'. Chapter 6 explored the women-abusing potential of existing childcare law, the structure and organization of childcare agencies, and childcare policies and procedures.

All of the abuses and potential abuses mentioned in this journey through childcare systems, have actually occurred. They are not aberrations; on the contrary, their nature and origin are such that they occur repeatedly, and often become permanent features of the agency and personnel in question. Thankfully, no woman is likely to endure all these abuses at any one time; but some of the abuses, separately, are so devastating in their impact, that women and children may never really recover. Actual case histories will be used in later chapters to convey the precise detail of these abuses and the consequences for mothers, children, professionals and their agencies.

PART II

Manifestations

7

The abuse of power: common experiences for workers and clients

Introduction

This book deals with the abuse of women in the context of childcare work. Childcare systems are not the only instrument of abuse of women. Abuse of women is widespread. The women most vulnerable to abuse by childcare systems are usually those who are disadvantaged and already experiencing different types of abuse. In many cases the problems which focus the attention of childcare workers on these mothers have their roots in deprivation, poverty and isolation. Women are often powerless in these situations. Many are isolated, stigmatized, single parents with more than one child. Often they do not have a stable, mutually supportive relationship with another adult but instead may even suffer abuse at the hands of an adult partner. These experiences are not unknown to childcare workers themselves, most of whom are women.

The basis for much of the abuse perpetrated against women, clients as well as workers, lies in the imbalance of and in the abuse of power. We will therefore begin with a definition of power. We will then explore this imbalance of power and some of the abuses arising from it. We will look, for example, at sexual harassment, domestic violence and rape, often perpetrated against women by their own partners. A number of case examples, taken from clients as well as workers, will be used to illustrate the arguments.

What is power?

It is often said that much of the abuse of women has its roots in power imbalance between men and women (Beale 1986; French 1993; Guerin

1994). But what exactly is meant by 'power'? What do we actually mean when we use phrases like 'power imbalance' or 'abuse of power'? This question is not easily answered. The main criteria for power is the ability to control others, the ability to get others to do things you want them to do. Within this definition power means different things to different people: a teacher has power over pupils; older pupils over younger ones; an employer has power over employees; an employee, for example, a bus driver, over passengers; a prime minister has power over citizens; a citizen, for example, a childcare worker, has power over parents. Power is relative. The term 'power' is, therefore, best understood as another word for 'control'.

People in positions of power are able not only to control other people, but they are also able to control whatever is necessary to achieve economic, social and psychological freedom and independence; this may include controlling information, money or health. People in positions of power are able to make sure that they themselves attain these things sufficiently. They are also in a position of control when, where and how others, in less powerful positions, can attain these things. Politicians are a perfect example of people in power in this sense. The problem is that they often forget that the votes of the 'powerless' actually give them these powers. Women clients who come into contact with childcare systems are usually not in positions of power in relation to the workers. They are usually not in a position to control the workers' behaviour, in fact they are usually the ones who are being controlled.

Power imbalance

The relationship between women clients and childcare workers is characterized by an imbalance of power. Power imbalance between workers and clients is intrinsic in the structure of the childcare system (see Chapters 5 and 6). Often, the worker has control and the client is being controlled. For example, if children are taken into care the workers set the criteria for their return home. These criteria may include changes in the client's behaviour or changes in her living arrangements. For example, the client may be asked to change her lifestyle, stay at home, drink less, or have different boyfriends. She may be asked to ensure that others change their behaviour, for example, that her husband or boyfriend moves out, if he has perpetrated child abuse, or that she ensures that her children return home at a certain time at night, or attend school. In either case, the worker usually has the power to control her, tell her what to do, and decide on the consequences of her behaviour.

Power is generally distributed along hierarchical lines. However, it is also distributed along gender lines (Reynolds 1986). Women are usually in positions of less power then men – we have looked at some of the reasons for this in Chapter 3. Traditionally women were dependent on their husbands or partners, economically as well as socially. In some cases women established their own support networks (Ridd and Callaway 1986). For example, within extended families women supported each other practically as well as emotionally. However, economically their male partners were usually in positions of power in relation to them. This has not changed much. Today men still tend to hold economic power in many families. For example, 70 per cent of British husbands do not discuss with their partners how much they earn. Although in other countries these figures are considerably lower (40 per cent in Germany and 1 per cent in the United States (Oakley 1982)), economic dependence of wives means that men control the family economically. Consequently, there is a power imbalance between husbands and wives when it comes to financial decision making. Inequality in the relationship often leads to the abuse of power.

Abuse of power

Power imbalance in itself does not have to lead to abuse. As we have seen, it can actually be used to prevent abuse, as is the case when child abuse is uncovered and powerful agencies act to protect children. Similarly, in most families the relationship between parents and children reflects power imbalance; however, as a rule this is aimed at protecting the children from harm or guiding them in their development. Power imbalance becomes abusive when people in power are no longer acting in the best interest of those with less power or when they respond violently to challenges to their own position. Examples abound. When power is challenged, parents may resort to punishing their children physically, governments resort to military action, childcare workers resort to removing children into care. Sexual harassment, domestic violence and rape are typical examples of gender related abuse of power. All of these manifestations of power abuse are experienced by childcare workers as well as clients.

Sexual harassment

Sexual harassment is one of the most common forms of abuse of power. Both men as well as women, can be sexually harassed and the gender of the perpetrator does not necessarily have to be different from that of the abused. However, in the majority of cases sexual harassment is experienced by women and perpetrated by men. Gordon (1990) identified some of the reasons: 'cultural expectations about *women's sexuality*, the conception of them as objects and men as subjects, the vulnerability of women evident in sexual harassment, wife battering and rape, constitute a straitjacket on women expressing their sexuality' (p. 17).

Like so many other forms of power abuse, sexual harassment is not always obvious to the onlooker. It can be subtle and covert. Sometimes it is difficult to distinguish between covert sexual harassment and overtly friendly behaviour. Physical proximity or physical contact, for example, can be similar in both situations. In most cases, however, the difference soon becomes apparent. Overtly friendly behaviour is usually experienced as pleasant and welcomed, while victims of covert sexual harassment usually experience the advances as inappropriate and unwanted. Myers (1993) emphasized that, 'these acts are anchored by the effects on the victim ... and not by the intent of the perpetrator' (p. 83). Overt sexual harassment is more clearly defined; it may include overt unwanted physical or verbal sexual approaches, such as inappropriate touching, hugging or kissing (we will deal with issues regarding rape later in this chapter), bribery or coercion ('If you want the promotion, you know what you have to do').

Sexual harassment in the workplace

Childcare workers as well as clients may experience sexual harassment in the work place. There is a clear definition and legal framework regarding overt sexual harassment. The European Commission's Recommendation defines it as 'unwanted conduct of a sexual nature or other conduct based on sex affecting the dignity of women and men at work' (Equal Opportunities Commission 1993: 4). Legally, sexual harassment can be challenged through the Equal Opportunities Commission.

An example from a fully qualified childcare worker helps to illustrate the effects of sexual harassment:

> On my first day in the Family and Childcare field work office I was welcomed by a team of five workers, three male and two female. This was a surprisingly high percentage of male workers for a family and childcare team; what was not surprising was that the senior social worker was one of the males. I had come from a residential setting in which gender issues had not been a problem and was really looking forward to the new work experience. The covert sexual harassment from the field workers came therefore as an unexpected surprise. It took me some time to figure out what was going on. It started off with the middle-aged senior social worker greeting me with a hug. While I did not think that this was very professional, I thought no more of it. Maybe it was just his way of wanting to make me feel welcome. I saw that some of the other female childcare workers seemed to enjoy this type of attention. At one point, when we met for multidisciplinary work, I heard a health visitor asking him 'Where is my hug?' It seemed that he saw nothing wrong with his behaviour and I did not want to be blamed for being oversensitive. However, soon his questions became intrusive. Did I have a

boyfriend? Was I sexually experienced? Did I want to get married? Did I want children? How did I feel towards my own sexuality? At first, I was surprised by these questions and did answer some of them. Soon, the two other male social workers joined in. There was jeering when I left the office, silence when I entered; there were deliberately discriminatory remarks 'just to get you going', there were derogatory comments. This went on until the senior left the office three years later. At times I wished he would have stepped over the mark, so that I could have taken him up in court. However, this never happened. What did happen was that, while I was highly qualified to work in the sensitive area of therapeutic intervention in child sex abuse and had done so very effectively, I was no longer allocated such cases.

This example is not an isolated incident (Wise and Stanley 1990). Myers (1993) used the phrase 'gender harassment' for similar situations when people engage in insulting and degrading sexist statements and behaviour. These situations are frequently typified by sexual innuendo, a 'boys club atmosphere' (French 1993), sexually explicit pictures of women on walls or in newspapers or advertising. The above example shows the abusing effect of such harassment on the worker: 'To a victim, the effects of discrimination or harassment may be pivotal to a career and are often devastating to one's personhood' (Myers 1993: 84).

Only a few women report sexual harassment in the workplace to the police. They are clear about the implications – 'its his word against mine'. Temporary or part-time workers are particularly vulnerable because they have even less protection than women in full-time and permanent jobs. Sexual harassment in the workplace does not only affect the people who experience it directly. It has indirect side effects. Victimized workers are usually preoccupied with the harassment and in turn unable to concentrate fully on their jobs. If childcare workers experience sexual harassment in the workplace, they themselves and their clients suffer. Most of the childcare clients are women in already vulnerable positions. Sexual harassment of childcare workers can, therefore, indirectly lead to increased abuse of women clients.

Sexual harassment at home

Most women clients of childcare workers are, in fact, not employed outside the home. They are looking after their children on a full-time basis. We have seen that clients may be indirectly affected if their childcare worker experiences sexual harassment because the worker's experiences of harassment in the office impinges on her ability to concentrate on her job. But do clients themselves also experience sexual harassment directly? Of course they do. Many of them are young, single mothers, living alone with their children, without adequate social support. They are easy targets for sexual harassment and intimidation. They become victims of sexual harassment in housing estates, in shopping malls, during leisure activities, in their own home.

Sexual harassment and gender

Sexual harassment does not only happen to women. It is not only perpetrated by men. Men can also be sexually harassed and the gender of the harassing person does not necessarily have to be different from that of the harassed: 'Sexual harassment is one means by which those who are not heterosexual males can be effectively subordinated, and is a widely used though often unrecognised form of violence' (Ramazanoglu 1987: 65). However, in most cases women are sexually harassed by men. The reason for this and, at the same time, the essence of sexual harassment was captured by Wise and Stanley (1990) who said that 'although the medium through which sexual harassment gets done is often "sex", actually its essence is power rather than sexuality' (p. 15).

Domestic violence

Another symptom of power abuse known to clients as well as childcare workers is domestic violence. Women's Aid, a movement offering refuge accommodation, support and advice to battered women and their children, defines domestic violence as 'the intentional and persistent mental or sexual abuse of a woman, or women and children, in a way that causes pain or injury or the threat of such abuse by her male partner with whom she lives or has lived' (McMinn 1991: 10). The words of a childcare worker, who experienced domestic violence herself, describe the impact of this type of abuse:

> I left my husband four months before my twenty-first wedding anniversary. I had made one attempt five years before that, but returned home after three weeks. I had nowhere else to go with the children. We had married after a whirlwind romance, and I had found myself pregnant. Marriage was the only choice that I could morally make at that time, in 1970. We scarcely knew each other. I had been a girl of many talents, university graduate, top of the class in many subjects, and a good athlete, independent in personality and popular with all. Loving and much loved.
>
> My life changed rapidly. We had two children within the year. The upsets seriously started when he could not get himself up in the morning. He would smash crockery off the wall, use appalling language. One day, I do not remember much more, except to say that I had just finished knitting a yellow jersey. I proudly put it on, for the first time. I thought he would like it. He punched me in the face. I got a bloody nose. The red blood seeped into my new yellow jumper. I was stunned, shocked. I was sore. That's when the serious violence began: thumping and hitting and kicking and smacking and

punching. Even when I was with child, he punched me in the stomach. I thought I was going to lose the child.

I did not have a clue how to respond. Given my own sheltered childhood, I had not believed that someone like himself could even exist. He said, that it was my fault, that I was inadequate. Maybe he was right. I tried harder. I wanted to please him. I blamed myself for his attacks. But the violence continued. Most of the time, I curled up and just hoped for the best. The years rolled on. I was trapped in every way, or so it seemed. Eventually, I fell ill and was forced into medical retirement. I was in very deep despair. I went to the so-called professionals for help. No one had time for me. They were wasting my time, and I theirs. I concluded that no one could help me, a hard hitting thing for a sick person. I left. He stayed in the family home. I had to find a flat for me and the kids.

A few, dear friends gave me a leg up. No judgement regarding my sad behaviour, no devastating attacks, only concern. Today, three years and several moves later, I know, I am getting better. I have again a lovely home and my children are easy in my company.

This report comes from a well educated, professional women. At the time when she experienced domestic violence neither her colleagues nor her friends knew what was going on behind closed doors. She was eventually able to leave and make a new start. She is not the only one. Women clients as well as childcare workers experience this kind of domestic violence.

The prevalence of domestic violence

The problem of domestic violence was not openly brought to people's attention until, in the 1970s, the Women's Aid movement was established. Legally, domestic violence was recognized as a problem in England with the introduction of the Domestic Proceedings and Magistrates' Court Act (1976) (Quinn 1991). It is still difficult to assess the exact prevalence of domestic violence. Research findings vary considerably and depend on the methodology used (Oakley 1982). However, it is evident that marriage is not a precondition for domestic violence (McLaughlin *et al.* 1992) and that although domestic violence is experienced in all social groups (Robinson 1991) people in lower socioeconomic groups are particularly vulnerable (Connors *et al.* 1992). Women clients of childcare workers are often not married and usually come from lower socioeconomic groups. They are, therefore, particularly vulnerable.

Reporting domestic violence

Research figures are obviously based on reported incidence of domestic violence. The real figure is probably much higher. One of the main reasons why domestic violence is not reported is fear (McMinn 1991). Ironically women have more to fear from the men they love than from strangers. Six times more violent acts are perpetrated against women by intimates than by strangers (French 1993). As Oakley (1982) put it: 'the state both supports the asymmetry of husband–wife relationships and ultimately condones male domestic violence by taking less notice of a man beating his wife behind even an open door than almost any other violent crime' (p. 258).

Another reason for under-reporting was identified by Quinn (1991) of the Northern Ireland Solicitors Family Law Association. She recognized that women who report domestic violence and seek protection will experience solicitors, courts, police, public and voluntary housing agencies and social services. Many of these agencies may be encountered for the first time. Quinn pointed out that these agencies and services are not always well coordinated: 'Each of us may be guilty to a certain extent of dealing with each aspect of the problem in an isolated and singular fashion' (1991: 22). Furthermore, these agencies are often unable to offer adequate protection. As recently as ten years ago police officers were taught to respond to reports of domestic violence by simply separating the parties involved and then leaving the scene (Connors *et al.* 1992). Police training was geared towards reconciliation rather than intervention (Donnan 1991). More recently the police training manual was updated and now recommends 'dealing with domestic assaults as criminal behavior, regardless of whether they occur in the home or elsewhere' (Connors *et al.* 1992: 322).

Even when incidents of domestic violence are reported, adequate response cannot be guaranteed. The public, including police and social services are reluctant to interfere because domestic violence is still widely viewed as a personal problem (French 1993). Superintendent Cyril Donnan (1991) confirmed that 'the police have an exaggerated respect for the closed doors of the family citadel' (p. 26). Oakley (1982) exposed this misconception:

> it is false to see the problem in individualistic terms. It is not individual men whose psychic structure turns them against individual women in a moment of temporary and understandable aberration. Physical force and its threat used against women by men in marriage is a form of collective social control ... of a dominant group keeping its subordinates in line. (p. 255)

Hanmer and Statham (1988) agree that domestic violence is not just an illustration of patterns of individual relationships but 'the expression of a system of stratification in which differential status is an emergent property of the distribution of power' (p. 81). Horley (1990) elaborated: 'the root of the problem lies in society itself ... Critical to this is the realisation that the fundamental problem is not battering but men's abusive power over women' (p. 16).

The cycle of domestic violence

Once domestic violence has become part of family life, it is difficult to break the cycle. Most women do not talk about domestic violence. Donnan (1991) found that women are assaulted up to 35 times before they report domestic violence to the police. Most women try and deal with it within the four walls of their own home. They blame themselves for the abuse and try and change their behaviour to suit their partner and thus avoid his anger. This strategy usually only works for a short period of time, then violence continues. In the first instance women tend to seek help from family or friends (Donnan 1991). When women approach outside agencies they usually turn to the family doctor first. At this point they may be treated for minor injuries or depression, anxiety or nervousness. They may even be admitted to psychiatric hospitals (Hanmer and Statham 1988). When they approach the police their case is often dealt with by young officers who are reluctant to get involved (Donnan 1991).

Few women leave their partners permanently after the first incident of domestic violence. Some seek temporary shelter, support or protection either with friends or in a refuge. Many return within days or weeks. McMinn (1991) outlined the reasons for this: fear, economic dependence, guilt, loss of confidence due to the violence, his promises to change, trying to keep the family together, and lack of support from professionals. Oakley (1982) recognized that 'men's right to keep their wives in order by any means they choose is another item on the covert agenda of sexual relations behind the tempting fantasy of the romantic idyll' (p. 256).

Women tend to remain in the cycle of domestic violence. However, when violence turns against their children many women leave. Refuge workers are familiar with the following kind of statement: 'My own abuse was bad enough but I could handle it. Sometimes I blamed myself for making him mad. Maybe I was not good enough. But when he started hitting my daughter I was ready to kill. That's when I left.' Childcare workers are aware of the cycle of domestic violence and treat these kind of statements with caution. While in many cases women do not return home after such incidents, women who return to their violent partners after he attacked the children are held responsible for not protecting their children. Again, the responsibility for the man's behaviour is placed firmly with the woman. Men are avoided by childcare workers, especially when they are violent (see Chapter 8).

Domestic violence and child abuse

There is evidence of a relationship between domestic violence and child abuse. Connors *et al.*'s (1992) research pointed to 'the lowest rates of child abuse among parents who did not hit one another, with high violence-prone husbands and wives the most likely child abusers' (p. 325). If hitting one another is part of the relationship pattern in a family, it does not have to reach crisis proportions to have negative side-effects (LaVigna and Donnellan 1986; Dillenburger and Keenan 1994a). Many children are hit, smacked, or slapped on a daily basis. In fact, this kind of domestic violence, that is, physical punishment, is widely accepted as a method in child rearing (Dillenburger and Keenan 1994a). Many people do not even consider smacking children child abuse. However, when physical violence is condoned in one situation, it is difficult to condemn it in another. When smacking young children is condoned, where do we draw the line? When does physical punishment become physical abuse? If the parent smacking the child is justified, is the man who hits his wife justified?

These questions lie at the root of the debate about domestic violence. Abusive partners often claim that their violent outbursts were caused by the behaviour of their spouse. They say that she deserved being hit because she was 'nagging; getting at me; not cleaning the house; or not having the dinner ready'. They feel justified in physically punishing her 'misbehaviour'. As we have seen in the example earlier many abused wives actually feel guilty for causing such outbursts. They accept blame for their husband's violent behaviour: 'If I had done what he wanted me to, he wouldn't have hit me.' This misconception leads to further abuse and the continuation of the cycle of domestic violence. Domestic violence whether perpetrated against children or adults is abusive. The role of childcare workers must be to prevent it.

Rape

Rape is the ultimate abuse of women. It is defined by law as: 'A man commits a rape if he has unlawful sexual intercourse with a woman who at the time of intercourse does not consent to it' (Sexual Offences (Amendment) Act 1976). The maximum penalty for the offence is life imprisonment (Offences Against the Person's Act 1861; Sexual Offences Act 1956). But is that what actually happens? Does society take rape as seriously as the law would have us believe? Obviously not, otherwise the number of rapes would decrease. That is not the case. In fact, cases of rape seem to be increasing. As Oakley (1982) put it, rape is viewed as:

an essentially 'normal' masculine enterprise, and apparently becoming more normal, as it is reported more and more often – a 100 per cent increase in London from the first quarter of 1977 to the first quarter of 1978, a steady rise in America from the early 1930s on, to a rate of one every nine minutes in 1976. (p. 261)

Experiencing rape

The experience of rape is difficult to capture in words. Women who have been raped say that the sheer panic, fear, feeling of powerlessness, worthlessness, dirtiness, guilt, and abuse that they experienced during and after the rape are beyond description. Rape is the most extreme abuse of power and victims are often unable to talk about their experience for many years to come. A professional foster parent, who had agreed that her experience of rape could be included in this book was, in the end, unable to report her story to the authors. Despite the fact that anonymity was obviously guaranteed she was overwhelmed by the pain of the memories each time she begun to talk about her rape. In her place we recite a poem by Marge Piercy in which the experience of rape is described:

Missoala Rape Poem

There is no difference between being raped
and being pushed down a flight of cement steps
except that the wounds also bleed inside.

There is no difference between being raped
and run over by a truck
except that afterwards men ask you if you enjoyed it.

There is no difference between being raped
and losing a hand in a mowing machine
except that doctors don't want to get involved,
the police wears a knowing smirk,
and in small towns you become a veteran whore.

There is no difference between being raped
and being bitten on the ankle by a rattlesnake
except that people ask if your skirt was short
and why were you out alone anyhow.

There is no difference between being raped
and going head first through a windshield
except that afterward you are afraid
not of cars
but of half the human race.

Response to rape

Similar to domestic violence, statistics on rape depend on reported cases. Connors *et al.* (1992) observed that 'rape is significantly under-reported by victims due to the stigma associated with a sexual crime, possible insensitive police responses, and the trauma of a public trial or guilt over failure to prevent rape' (p. 322).

The public response to rape is two-fold. On the one hand, there is still an assumption that rape victims must have somehow provoked the attack. Public images of women in short skirts or low cut tops are used to entice people into buying cars, holidays, aftershave, showerlotions, etc. If women dress this way in real life, they are told that they only have themselves to blame if they are sexually assaulted or raped. Even if they were not dressed this way, they stand accused if they were raped; maybe they were out late at night alone, or went for a walk alone in a park or forest. In these cases, the responsibility for sexual assault and rape is placed firmly on the victim rather then the perpetrator. Sexual assault and rape of women (or young girls, in cases of child sex abuse) are probably the only crimes where this type of argument is so frequently used, that many women begin to believe it themselves and experience feelings of guilt and self-blame after the attack.

On the other hand, public awareness of the issues involved in sexual assault and rape has risen over the past few years. Increasingly support is available to victims. Voluntary support groups offer confidential counselling and help. The police have established procedures which are much more sensitive to the needs of rape victims than they had been in the past. For example, women police officers are available to establish special relationships with rape victims and to offer support throughout the proceedings.

While this is a step in the right direction, it still places the responsibility of dealing with rape with women. The difference is that now the victim as well as the prosecutor are female. Men seem to be out of the picture, exonerated of any responsibility. However, rape is also abusive to men. Most men do not rape women and are horrified and appalled at the fact that some do. In order to tackle the full impact of rape on women as well as men, the underlying issue needs to be addressed. The reason why women are raped is not that men cannot control their sexual drives, or that women dress provocatively, it is the unequal stratification of power between men and women.

Date rape and rape in marriage

Responses to date rape or marital rape are ambiguous. In many American states marital rape is still legal (French 1993). Recently, date rape has become a highly publicized phenomenon, particularly in cases occurring at prestigious colleges (French 1993). The problem is at least two-fold. First, as in most rape cases, there are usually no outside witnesses. Second, in public perception dating and sexual intercourse are nearly synonymous. Consequently, a women who dates is expected to consent to sex. If she does not, the man cannot be blamed for misinterpreting her protest. Given this misleading perception, it is not surprising that convictions for date rape are infrequent.

Similar circumstances are present in cases of marital rape. With the marriage vow, it is presumed that both parties consent to sex as part of their relationship. In fact, in the past it was deemed the man's right to have sex with his wife. So much so that the marriage certificate offered immunity to perpetrators of sexual assault and rape (French 1993). Today, however, after much debate the Law Commission (1992) recommended that 'there is no marital immunity in the crime of rape' (p. 11) and suggested a minimum penalty of five years' imprisonment.

The relationship to the perpetrator and the effects of rape

Some may think that being raped by someone you know must be less traumatic than being raped by a stranger. In fact, research evidence does not support such a view. Research into the psychological effects of rape has shown that there are virtually no differences between women who have been raped by their husband, by dates or by strangers (Riggs *et al.* 1992). Data for the subjective and objective danger of the attack, depressive episodes, social phobia, or sexual dysfunction were similar for all victim groups. In regard to other diagnostic criteria rape victims were more vulnerable then women in non-victimized control groups. Researchers concluded that 'complete rape, regardless of the victim's relationship to the perpetrator, is a traumatising experience that may lead to psychological difficulties' (Riggs *et al.* 1992: 286).

The Law Commission (1992) seemed to take this type of research into account. In fact, they recommended that marital rape should be considered as an offence as serious or even more serious than rape by a stranger: 'it is accepted that child sex abuse is at its most wicked when perpetrated within the family; perhaps the same reasoning should apply to attacks on adult members' (p. 9).

Reporting marital rape

Being raped by a person with whom one has an ongoing relationship, be it in marriage, cohabitation, or dating is probably an experience many women have in common. It is difficult to obtain exact figures about the prevalence of this type of rape for a number of reasons. First, marital rape, like other forms of rape, is still highly stigmatizing. Second, women are traumatized by the experience of rape and consequently are unable to report it. Third, if women prosecute their own husband for marital rape they most likely have to leave him. As we have seen earlier, women who are caught in the cycle of violence cannot to do this.

Reported data show that about 10 per cent of women experience marital rape at some time in their lives. Since marital rape is a particular kind of domestic violence, it is not surprising that the prevalence is higher for battered wives. Research indicates that as many as 30–50 per cent of women in refuges or shelters for battered wives have been raped by their husbands. Marital rape is much less likely (1–4 per cent) in non-abusive relationships (Riggs *et al*. 1992).

Conclusion

Women, clients as well as workers, experience different forms of gender related abuse of power. Sexual harassment, domestic violence and rape were discussed in this context. These kinds of abuse are detrimental not only to the person who experiences them herself but also the people with whom she has contact, especially if they depend on her for their care. Clients often depend on the care of workers, consequently clients will suffer when workers are abused. Children depend on the care of an adult, usually their mother, consequently children will suffer when mothers are abused. Women clients of childcare agencies are therefore doubly vulnerable. They are vulnerable to the abuse by childcare systems as well as to the abuse from powerful others in their lives. Exact figures of the extent to which women are abused do not exist. However, childcare workers dealing with women clients must be aware that their women clients may have abusive experiences apart from those directly obvious. Women often do not disclose the abuse they suffer until their children are directly affected. For example, many women do not leave their partner even if he batters them regularly. However, when he batters the children, women usually leave.

Abuse such as that perpetrated within an abusive childcare system can only augment their problems. The following chapter will concentrate on manifestations of such abuse. Concrete case examples will be given of abuse perpetrated during the various stages of childcare investigation and intervention.

8

Abuse in action

Introduction

This chapter will focus upon abusive practices in each phase of childcare work. These phases are: referral, investigation, emergency protection through intervention, case conference, care proceedings, assessment, fostering, and adoption. It will use case material accumulated in the authors' own experiences and research, and, in the experiences of practitioner and academic colleagues. The first case chosen will illustrate specific abuses against a mother during the referral and investigation phase. Additional cases will be used for the same purpose in subsequent phases. The context of the abuse will be highlighted. This will give some indication of the underlying causes and motivation of those who are abusing. They may or may not be aware of the abuses they perpetrate, but their behaviour constitutes abuse nevertheless. Reference will be made throughout the chapter to the content of earlier chapters in which possible causes and motivation were explored in depth.

Referral

The abuse of women by childcare professionals often begins during the referral phase of childcare work. The reason is simple: referral taking is a complex and difficult task for which childcare workers receive little or no formal training (O'Hagan 1989). Workers are often unaware of the potentially abusive attitudes with which they approach the task, and of many characteristics in the referral-taking situation, and within the childcare system in which they work, which will encourage those attitudes to become manifest. A very common abuse of women occurs when they ask an agency for help, such as financial assistance, or refuge from domestic violence; during the interview, the worker finds reason to convert the original referral into one of child protection; the woman is not informed. In one of the author's experiences as a Principal Case Worker in Child Protection (and in the evidence of research: see Chapter 6), referrals about children of single parent mothers predominated. The following referral is typical.

> Two neighbours contact social services to allege that Maureen, a 19 year old single parent, is leaving her two children John, aged 3, and Christine, aged 8 months, with a new boyfriend, on numerous nights in the week, and that this boyfriend has been known to beat the children. The neighbours can give no further information about the case; they do not know the name of the new boyfriend. They say that Maureen has just recently moved into the area; but they are adamant that the children are being abused. The worker is worried by this referral and feels that it should be investigated as soon as possible. Her senior agrees.

This is an inadequate referral and contains many potentially abusive interpretations. A literal acceptance of everything said on the referral may indicate a generally abusive attitude; abusive (mis)interpretations stemming from that attitude may include the following:

> Another referral involving a single parent mother! These children are being doubly abused; their mother is not there, and they're being minded by somebody totally unfit for the job. The mother must know this; the kids must be distressed when she returns. Mother is responsible whether she knows or not. It needs substantiating by seeing the children; we need to see the children, or speak to some professional, preferably a health visitor or GP, to verify; we could ask a health visitor who knows the family, to visit, or we could check to see if she's attending a nursery, and get some information there. We need to move quickly: these kids are in danger.

Many aspects of childcare training and many components within the childcare system facilitate this kind of stigmatizing and scapegoating. For example, the training of workers is likely to have been dominated by those developmental and child rearing theories inevitably leading to the view that mothers are responsible for the abuse of their children, irrespective of who perpetrates the abuse. Some professionals may contribute to the prevailing anti-single parent climate; they may hold genuine convictions about young single parents' irresponsibility (as many politicians and moralists already do), and regard them as the 'major social problem of our time'. Their caseloads are likely to be dominated by multi-problem single parent families in which they see no prospect of change or improvement. In the light of some recent enquiry report, detailing the horrific death of a child by the partner of a single parent (the most common happening in past reports), the managers of childcare agencies may have generated anxiety among staff by issuing warning memos about the need to take this kind of referral seriously, and to act promptly. The manager will remind staff of the 'strict procedures' in operation. The worker may take very seriously the department's (and the Children Act's) emphasis upon the welfare of the child being paramount, and may genuinely feel (even at this early stage) that the welfare of these children is being dangerously neglected; additionally, the worker may be one of those who believes that the welfare of the child and the rights of a single parent mother in a referral situation such as this, are incompatible (a view possibly strengthened by numerous personal and/or professional experiences in the past). This may fuel the intent to investigate without the mother knowing, or getting another professional to surreptitiously investigate on their behalf.

Anonymous referrals

There is even more likelihood of this kind of thinking and attitude when the referral is anonymous. An anonymous referral presents the most difficult referral-taking task. It can quickly trap the worker in a double bind: the referrer may insist that he/she be asked no questions, yet the referral necessitates many questions; the worker will desperately want to 'hold onto the referrer', yet sense that the referrer will put the phone down at the merest hint of any enquiry about identity or location. Anonymous referrals often provoke a crisis for the worker, which adversely impacts upon the attempt to make a professional response, increasing whatever risks there are of unprofessional, potentially abusive, thinking and attitude in referral-taking generally.

Investigation

A sound, comprehensive referral necessitates either an 'investigation' or an 'assessment'. These two terms are often used synonymously, and should not be. The Department of Health (1988) makes a clear distinction between them. Assessment is a much more elaborate and time consuming task than that of investigation. Investigation is the second phase of child protection work, after referral. Assessment will be necessary at a later stage of child protection when there is more time and less pressure on workers. Let us for the moment concentrate on investigation, using the same case as in the referral phase above.

> The social worker checks to see if the mother is known to social services. She is. There is a long history of involvement going back to when the mother herself was in care, as a consequence of her being physically and sexually abused by her stepfather. Numerous anonymous allegations similar to the present one have been made and have been investigated. The worker contacts a local health visitor named in the records, and discusses the case

with her. She is given additional information about the children; their physical development is OK. She provides the name of a nursery John is attending. The worker visits the nursery and speaks to staff. They introduce her to John. He is busily engaged in play. She attempts to talk to him about home, but he is not interested. School staff talk about Maureen in terms of 'she's only a child herself ... gets herself into all kinds of bother'. They make the point that they are reasonably happy with John's progress. They have observed no indications of physical punishment, though they say he sometimes comes to the nursery full of anxiety and tension, and it takes him a while to settle and unwind. The worker returns to the office and contacts the police. The police inform her that they do know the family; they have been called out on a number of occasions to the home, because of complaints of rowdiness; no action was taken. They know nothing about the new boyfriend. Later that day, a social worker and police officer visit the home.

These developments may appear to be necessary and professional – that is, a worker's rigorous attempts to gain as much knowledge as possible before visiting. But, similar to the referral phase, certain women-abusing characterisitics are emerging. First, the preoccupation with the woman and her childcaring, to the virtual exclusion of any interest in her male partner, ironically, the alleged abuser. No one knows anything about him of course, but that is the likely consequence of previous preoccupations with Maureen and previous disinterest in or avoidance of her male partners. Second, the visit to the school and the attempt to use 3 year old John for information gathering constitutes a serious abuse of both mother and child. Third, the social worker has made contact with police, health visitor and school staff, and made numerous enquiries about Maureen and her children without Maureen knowing anything about it. This means that perceptions, intuitions, assessments, decision making and judgements, all of which have been made in the past, have been resurrected to enlighten and to help professionals in the present. They may all be relevant and accurate; but there is also the possibility that they may not be. What is indisputable is that they will influence the approach and attitude of the professionals given the task of visiting the home in response to the referral.

Investigative visit

The social worker and police officer choose to visit at around 4 p.m. They wish to see the children and also speak to Maureen alone. They calculate (rightly) that her boyfriend will not be at home at 4 p.m. Maureen recognizes them immediately, and is angered. 'What is it this time?' she asks. They tell her. She manages to control a powerful sense of anger and resentment building up inside her. 'Those bastards across the road!' she says, alluding to someone she thinks has made the referral. But she has been here before, and knows that they will tell her nothing about the identity of the referrer. They ask her has she been leaving her children in the care of a stranger.

'An' what of it?' she replies.

'Did you know he had beaten them?'

'Who says?'

'They were heard screaming.'

'They're screaming all the time; if ye stay long enough, you'll hear them.'

Here the workers are not only abusing Maureen in the most obvious sense, but they are making it virtually impossible to carry out a comprehensive and professional investigation. Their approach is accusatory and interrogative, yet based upon an allegation that someone other than Maureen has abused the children. Their approach conveys the view that they hold Maureen responsible for whatever happens to the children, be she present or absent. This accusatory, interrogative approach has its origins in the file records on Maureen, and on colleagues' perceptions and feelings about her. It also stems to some extent from a fixation on the principle that the welfare of the child is paramount; this is the matter which dominates to the exclusion of everything else. Note that no attempt has yet been made to explore why Maureen left her children with a male friend, whether or not there were reasonable grounds for doing so, or indeed, if she had any choice in the matter. Nor as yet are there questions about difficulties she may be facing in life generally.

Deception and manipulation

One of the social workers tries to engage both the children. Eight month old Christine is crawling about on the floor. John is at the table playing with some Sticklebrick. The social worker moves between both children, smiling, talking, and touching, and getting closer to each of them. Maureen realizes, and says contemptuously:

'Why don't you ask me if they've got bruises?'

The social worker pretends to ignore Maureen. Her colleague asks:

'How often does this friend mind your children?'

'As often as I ask him?'

'How often's that?'

'Twice a week?'

The social worker 'playing' with the children spots some tearing of the skin behind John's ears. She draws Maureen's attention to it and asks if she knew anything about it. Maureen is extremely agitated at this point. She had not noticed this tearing before. She lifts John away from the social worker. John protests vigorously. Maureen shouts at him and tries to look at the back of his ears. She is angry and embarrassed. 'Who did that?' she asks, in a tone combining threat and defence. The threat is directed at John, whom she holds responsible for not telling her about this, thus leaving her vulnerable (and defensive) to this investigation, which she detests. She knows that they will now want to look at both children with their clothes removed, and then have them seen by a paediatrician. She will protest vehemently, but she realizes that they will do as they wish in the end.

Here again, the abuse of women is obvious and inevitable, given the nature of the initial contact. The workers have trapped themselves in their preoccupation with whether or not the children have been abused by some male stranger. They must pursue this enquiry. But they choose to do so surreptitiously (pretending to want to play with the children), which can only provoke Maureen further. There are many occasions when a mother will not realize the manipulative techniques of investigating workers, but here they are so blatant, and the mother is so experienced that the investigative process is fast becoming a sham. The most serious abuse is that the actions of the workers are increasingly rendering Maureen incapable of healthy positive interactions with her children during their visit. Their behaviour exposes their conviction that she must be responsible for whatever happened; this is becoming reciprocated in Maureen's behaviour indicating that she holds the children responsible.

Finally, a word on the matter of childcare workers looking for indicators of abuse on a child's body. Looking at particular bruising on the arms, face and legs used to be a common occurrence in investigation, and, provided workers approached the parent honestly, tactfully and sensitively, did not cause too much offence. But the authoritarian drift in child protection work during the 1980s (King and Trowell 1992; Cooper 1993) had the effect of lessening tact and sensitivity, and demanded much more, as is indicated in Dale *et al.* (1986): 'seeing the child means seeing under the child's clothing. It is not sufficient to establish that there are no bruises or injuries to the face, legs and arms' (p. 47).

It is certainly desirable to know of whatever injuries have been inflicted upon children, but this implicit instruction from Dale *et al.*, which was accepted by many childcare professionals, is fraught with moral and professional implications (apart from the probability that it was a significant contributory factor in the spate of bogus social workers and health visitors who consequently descended upon single mothers in ever increasing numbers, demanding to see their children undressed. The problem was particularly rife in Leeds, compelling childcare authorities to issue a statement to the press declaring their staff had no right whatsoever to see children undressed, and advising parents to refuse any such request (Leeds City Council 1990)). The authors of this text believe that provided a primary carer freely and willingly consents, professionally qualified childcare workers, in possession of their authorization and identity cards, should see whatever injury the carer directs their attention to. *We do not believe that childcare workers have a right to see children undressed,* nor do we believe that they have the right to ask a carer to see a child undressed. If unseen injuries are suspected it will be the reponsibility of a doctor to confirm them.

Intervention

There are numerous forms of intervention: (1) medical examination; (2) a child protection order; (3) placing a child in alternative accommodation; (4) searching for the parents/carers of a child (that is, where children have been left alone or abandoned by carers); (5) issuing a warning or caution to carers; (6) convening a case conference; and (7) establishing community or statutory support for carers temporarily unable to care at the time a referral is being investigated. Some may regard a medical examination as a standard procedure in *investigation*, not intervention; but if you ask any parent/carer they will invariably (and justifiably) regard a medical as a massive intervention. Similarly, some may have difficulty seeing item 4 (which is very common in child protection work) as an intervention; but the reality is that launching a search and eventually finding parents/carers who have knowingly left their children at risk, again constitutes a significant (and necessary) intervention which will have numerous consequences for both agencies and family, not the least of which will be the crisis and confrontation when the professionals finally meet up with carers.

Parents generally, and single parent mothers in particular, may be abused during any of these differing forms of intervention. But in reality, it is single parent mothers in particular who are abused most frequently when childcare professionals:

1 carry out medical examinations without the mother being aware of it;
2 carry out medical examinations without the mother being present;
3 discuss results of medical examinations with the GP or the paediatrician without the mother being present;
4 fail to explain to a mother the legal obligation to intervene and the legal basis of any proposed removal of the child;
5 do not discuss with the mother the possibility of placing the child with approved friends or relatives rather than removal;
6 do not inform the mother of the child's whereabouts when the child has been removed;
7 do not facilitate adequate contact between child and mother;
8 issue veiled threats to a mother who does not agree to the child being removed to alternative accommodation;
9 threaten a mother with the removal of her child if she does not get a suspected male abuser to leave;

10　marginalize the mother in the whole process of intervention, whatever
form that may take, making her feel like a victimized bystander.

Some of the abuses of women during intervention have already been
illustrated and explored both practically and theoretically in previous
chapters. We will now look at a child protection case in which the abuses of
a mother began (as usual) during the referral phase, got progressively
worse during the investigative phase and climaxed in the intervention
phase. The woman in this case is not a single parent mother, nor is she the
only one abused. Nor is it simply a case of the system abusing women; it is
more accurately the case of the system continuing and intensifying the
abuses of a mother already set in motion by her former spouse and his
partner.

> Marie is 4 years old. Her mother, Jean, aged 28, and her father, Kevin, aged
> 30, separated some time ago. Each of them married again. Jean's husband is
> Paul, aged 35. They both own and manage a successful restaurant. Kevin's
> wife is Sheila, aged 25.
>
> Jean and Kevin agreed on custody and contact. Jean had custody and
> Marie stayed with Kevin at weekends and longer periods when appropriate
> (for example, if Jean and Paul were on holiday). This arrangement was
> acceptable to all the parties.
>
> During some play and conversation with Marie one weekend, Sheila
> thought she detected allegations that Paul had been doing 'naughty things to
> her'. She conveyed this to Kevin. They discussed the matter and decided to
> take Marie to their GP. He examined her and referred her to a paediatrician.
> He (the paediatrician) examined her, noted some 'genital interference', said
> that sexual abuse was likely, and referred the case to social services. Social
> services visited and consulted with the paediatrician. They then referred the
> case to the police, and a joint visit by police officer and social worker was
> made to the home of Kevin and Sheila. They interviewed Marie, using
> anatomical dolls, drawing aids and various other methods. The child neither
> added to, nor clarified, the statements she had originally made to Sheila. They
> interviewed Sheila and Kevin at length, asking many questions about Jean
> and Paul in particular. A check was later made by police to see if Paul had any
> convictions. He hadn't. The nursery attended by Marie was approached to
> explore if there were any indicators of abuse in the child's behaviour in the
> classroom. There weren't.
>
> The social worker and police officer eventually visited Marie's mother Jean
> and her husband Paul, the alleged abuser. Before this visit took place, police,
> social services and paediatrician agreed that Marie should remain with Kevin
> and Sheila until investigations suggested otherwise. If Marie's mother
> protested and tried to get the child herself, an emergency order would be
> sought to stop her.
>
> Neither Jean nor Paul ever had any contact with social services before.
> Both were shocked; Jean was initially devastated and emerged at the end of
> the interview full of hatred and anger. They were interviewed both
> separately and together. Paul was interviewed for a much longer period. His

responses gave no grounds for suspicion. Jean's responses gave no indication that she was either aware of any abuse taking place, nor that she participated in any abuse. It was eventually decided that Marie could return to her mother, and that a child protection case conference be held. Jean's immediate action was to remove Marie from the nursery school in which she was happily placed, and to apply through her solicitor to have the contact with Kevin and Sheila drastically curtailed.

Although, as previously stressed, this is a case in which all parties suffer, it is obviously the child's mother who suffers infinitely more as a consequence of the way the investigation and intervention were conducted. So much of the investigation and intervention was being carried out without her knowing, that her only interpretation of events when she found out, was that a grand conspiracy between Sheila, Paul and the agencies had been created. And how did she find out? By the knock on the door, by stranger professionals, who, whatever effort they make to convey impartiality, conveyed the very opposite. They could do nothing other than sound and act *partially*, that is, question Jean and Paul at length on the grounds that they had already been pursuing an investigation, and, interviewing Sheila, Kevin, and Marie, on the basis of a suspicion that Paul had sexually abused the child.

It is not difficult to imagine the impact of this visit and the interrogations which followed; the knowledge for example that Marie's genital area had been medically examined by a GP and a paediatrician (both of whom happened to be male), on the basis of something she said to Sheila. Jean is the primary carer of Marie, and is now facing the prospect of people, particularly her ex-husband and his wife, perceiving her as someone who has chosen a child sexual abuse perpetrator in place of Kevin. What emerged in the case conference however, was something worse; she was interrogated on the basis of a suspicion that she may have known about the (alleged) abuse; worse still, that she may have facilitated it in some way (the collusive mother idea: see Chapter 5). Numerous other important points emerged from the case conference.

First, instead of immediately tackling the thorny problem of secrecy, suspicion and fear created by the allegation, the professionals compounded it and intensified the secrecy, suspicion and fear. Second, the professionals chose to ignore a mother's right to know about the suspicion that her daughter was being sexually abused, and that allegations were being made about her partner; this was on the basis of a judgement that it was not in the interests of the investigation and possible proceedings which might follow. (An attempt was made to argue that it was on the basis of a judgement that informing mother at the outset was not in the child's interests.) Third, there was no attempt made to assess the child's general health, that is, the emotional, social, psychological and educational life of the child. When the relevant professionals were invited to comment on these matters during the conference, they unanimously agreed that she was extremely healthy in all aspects of development, and that the quality of care provided by the primary carer – that is, the mother – was of the highest standard. There was general agreement that if the child was being sexually abused, it was highly likely that there would be some indicators of it in her social or emotional or psychological or educational functioning. No such indicators were discernible by any of the relevant professionals involved. Fourth, no attempt was made during the investigation to predict the long-term impact of any of the actions taken. Yet at the conference no one disputed that the professionals had:

1 inflicted a major trauma upon Jean, the mother;
2 adversely affected the quality of care Jean could provide for Marie at a time of crisis for both;
3 greatly undermined the marriage of Jean and Paul, creating enormous tension and suspicion between them;
4 damaged (probably irreparably) the relationship between the two couples;
5 ensured that contact between Marie and her father would henceforth be characterized by tension and resentment, in place of the mutual satisfaction and convenience with which previous contact was made – contact was likely to be substantially reduced in the future;
6 probably been responsible for (or, by virtue of their making contact and enquiry of the nursery school staff without the mother knowing, made a major contribution to) Jean's decision to remove Marie from a school in which she was well integrated and thriving;
7 compounded and intensified hostility and resentment among all the adult parties, to the extent of causing enormous confusion in Marie. She will have great difficulty understanding and coping with the fact that good, mutually respectful relationships, among adults upon whom she depended, have turned sour. She may accept blame for this new and painful situation; indeed, she could be wittingly or unwittingly punished by any of the adults. Either of these eventualities would be emotionally and psychologically damaging, and particularly so if her mother was the one who punished and blamed her.

The abuse of mothers during investigation and intervention can be catastrophic for children. In the above case, the child was not registered, nor should she have been. But registration was not a matter of importance for the mother; too much damage had already been done for the decision not to register to have any positive impact on her or any of the other parties.

Case conference

The child protection case conference is a long established administrative facility enabling childcare professionals to share information and make recommendations on current cases. Due to legislative and policy changes in recent years, Social Services, who normally convene case conferences, have been compelled to allow parents to attend. In the vast majority of cases, this usually means allowing *mothers* to attend (O'Hagan 1994b), because single parent mothers dominate child protection caseloads, and, men, whether they be husbands or cohabitees, have a deep-seated reluctance to attend any childcare professional gathering, and they are seldom encouraged to attend. The abuse of women during the case conference phase takes many forms. Some of these will now be explored, followed by a case example in which the convening of the conference itself constituted a serious abuse of the mother in question.

Parental attendance: partnership?

Allowing parents to attend case conferences is supposed to be an expression of the spirit of partnership between parents and childcare agencies, which the Government is attempting to foster. But this allowance is merely a sham of real partnership, for some obvious reasons. First, partnership depends on equality, which is non-existent. Any parent involved in a child protection case is likely to be substantially less educated, articulate and confident, than the key professional(s) in that case. In the case conference arena, when all these (comparatively) privileged professionals are together, and the single parent mother faces them alone, the inequality – the imbalance of power – is most striking. Even in getting to the conference, the lone single parent mother is greatly disadvantaged. She will often be expected to get there unaided (no small feat considering her contemplation of what awaits her); on arriving, she will most likely have to sit waiting until summoned to enter; when she does enter the conference, she will feel the stares of some 12–18 professionals sitting comfortably, most of whom she has never met before. She is not likely to have met the chair of the conference either (O'Hagan 1994b). She may or may not be introduced to the participants; and if she is, she is immediately likely to forget most of them, due to her apprehension.

Second, this inequality and imbalance has been greatly magnified by the expenditure of millions of pounds in preparing *the professionals* for parental attendance at case conference, and spending nothing at all, either in time or money, in preparing parents themselves. It is a huge irony, and a major abuse of parents (particularly lone single parents) that while professionals throughout the UK have been attending training workshops, studying the latest literature and research, watching training videos, all for the purpose of preparing them to be able to cope better with parental attendance(!), that the sum total of effort made to help parents cope with attendance has been nothing more than a chat with their social worker, in which they are informed of their right to attend. Little wonder that many parents do not accept the offer (Thoburn 1992; Bell 1993; O'Hagan 1994b).

Third, there is no real partnership in decision making, and the imbalance of power will quickly manifest itself when and if a parent disagrees with decisions and recommendations the professionals wish to make. As one parent in O'Hagan's research stated: 'I never saw myself in partnership with social services ... "partnership" is a bit over the top; social services always had the power'.

Variation in implementation of parental attendance policy

The partnership concept is further exposed in the enormous variations in the practice of parental attendance at case conferences. A particularly unpleasant practice is to ask the parent(s) to leave the conference at some point in order to enable professionals to discuss and to decide (Thoburn 1992; Bell 1993). The parent returns to hear what these decisions are and is invited to comment on them. Another practice is not to allow parents to attend the all important initial case conference, on the grounds that it would be too stressful for them (when in reality, it would be too challenging for the professionals). They are allowed to attend the subsequent review conference which take place three to six months later, but their attendence throughout the whole conference may again be at the discretion of the chair. Some authorities exclude parents from the decision making phases of all conferences; some chairpersons may permit the presence of a parent only for the purpose of informing them what the decisions were. It is perplexing to know that many childcare managers and professionals do not realize that such practices constitute the antithesis of parental participation and partnership. Single parent mothers are more vulnerable to, and more hurt by, such practices. The views of a parent in O'Hagan's research (when asked to leave the conference) surely represents the feelings of the majority of parents subjected to these practices: 'I felt betrayed; treated as a child'.

Case history

The decision to hold an initial case conference may be an abuse in itself. Reference was made in Chapter 6 to the potential abuse of rigid, all-embracing procedures put into effect in response to child abuse referrals. The following case demonstrates the abusive potential of unwarranted case conferences.

Margaret is a single parent, 20 years old, with two children, Ruth, aged 4, and Gemma, aged 18 months. She was cohabiting with John, 19 years old; he was the father of Gemma.

The couple row frequently; John leaves the home, and some weeks later, Ruth tells her mother that John did 'dirty things to her'. Margaret explores this with the child, and examines her genital and anal area. She is alarmed and incensed to see some indication of swelling and interference. She immediately takes Ruth to the police. The police interview Margaret at length. They seek to establish precisely when Ruth became aware of this, and whether or not she played any part in it, directly or indirectly. They arrange for Ruth *and Gemma* to be examined by a paediatrician. Margaret approves, and takes the children to the hospital. The paediatrician interviews Margaret at length too. He also wishes to explore a wider context beyond that of the suspected abuse – namely, Margaret's caring capacities, her own upbringing and, her relationship with the children. He confirms that Ruth has been sexually abused, but Gemma has not. He tells Margaret. She cannot control her feelings of anger and hatred for John. The paediatrician informs the hospital social workers, who inform the area social services office in the locality in which the family live. Margaret is interviewed by two social workers. The police search for John, without success. Margaret is asked many questions about herself, her relationships, upbringing, feelings and attitudes; they directly ask her, as the police, paediatrician and hospital social workers had done: has she ever been aware that this abuse was taking place. They conclude by informing her that a case conference will be held. Margaret feels humiliated and confused, and still very very angry. She is angry because of what John has allegedly done, and she repeatedly expresses a wish to kill him; but she is particularly confused and angry about the way she is being treated by professionals, the way she has been caught up in a spiralling bureaucratic process. The social workers consult with their senior; he consults with the area manager. A case conference is convened. When this is explained to Margaret, she erupts.

Margaret's feelings are understandable. She has acted responsibly throughout. She reported to the police immediately, and named the alleged perpetrator (perhaps risking some violent consequences). She willingly took the children for medical examinations (no small feat for a single parent mother traumatized by the discovery that her 4 year old had been sexually abused). She permitted the paediatrician to carry out a thorough medical examination, including detailed examination of the child's genitalia. She tolerated police officers, paediatrician, and social workers in two locations questioning her in depth about all manner of things. And for this, she is now to be subjected to a case conference in which professionals will consider whether or not to place her children's name on the child protection register (they could also decide more interventionist actions). She suffers a further indignity as a consequence of the investigation. Her own parents, a fiercely independent and strong willed couple, actually take over responsibility for the children, and compel Margaret to live with them. They also express disgust at developments, but remind Margaret of their repeated warnings about the character of John.

This type of abuse of women is very common. The reason is because the procedures and guidelines lack sophisticated criteria enabling workers and their managers to decide with confidence whether or not case conferences are necessary (see Chapter 5 on systems abuse). Typical of these criteria are the following, taken from the procedures of a number of authorities:

> A case conference shall be convened when following investigation there is considered to be substance to:
> - the allegation that a child is at risk of abuse;
> - the allegations that a child has been or is being abused;
> - the suspicions of abuse or if an element of doubt remains.

These criteria compel managers and frontline staff to convene many more conferences than are necessary. They say nothing about the type or degree of abuse, the location in which the abuse takes place, nor, the crucial factor about the identity of the perpetrator and his or her relationship with the child. Women like Margaret, entirely innocent of any abuse, who acted promptly in contacting the proper authorities, and who cooperated with them fully, at considerable cost to herself, deserve more sophisticated criteria than these. As a single parent mother, she suffered the additional humiliation of responsibility for her child being taken from her by her parents. Had her parents not done so, however, a worse fate may have occurred: a number of professionals actually suggested that Ruth be temporarily removed from her mother until such times as a comprehensive assessment be made. There was no consideration of the consequences of such a removal. When the intentions of the grandparents were made known, it was a source of relief to the professionals; no one considered the risks to Margaret's sense of worth and her future mothering capacities (see Chapter 5: 'grandmothers know best').

Care proceedings

Care proceedings contain more potentially abusive features than any other phase of childcare work. The vast majority of 'parents' subjected to abuses in care proceedings are women; they are likely to be single parent mothers, or, they may have husbands or partners who choose not to attend court, or who cannot attend. The mothers of children who are the subject of proceedings must attend. The following abuses of women are as diverse as they are common; they can be observed in court settings, in family proceedings, any day.

Location and atmosphere

Care proceedings take place in court. Often women have to wait hours in drab, smoke filled corridors of dilapidated Victorian buildings. Often they will be in close proximity to persons convicted or charged with all kinds of offences, attending other courts. They will later enter a court arena characterized by ritual and formality unfamiliar and challenging to them. They may have had sleepless nights worrying about these proceedings, and they may well be extremely agitated and apprehensive as they wait; yet their solicitor and social worker may have little time for them (the author recalls one occasion when as a guardian *ad litem*, on the day of a hearing, he finally caught up with the solicitor for the child; but the solicitor was dashing between two different courts dealing with four separate cases on the same day). Some observations will be incomprehensible to mothers as they sit waiting to be called; for example, social workers, guardians *ad litems*, police officers and solicitors (including their own solicitor), all talking to each other, friendly, bantering and joking with each other, gossiping about this and that and anything; the mother is here fighting to hold onto her child!

Adversarial court

No such niceties of professional camaraderie will be witnessed by mothers in the court. Here the professionals, predominantly male, become adversaries. The mother, and the quality of care she provides, is central to each of their submissions. The mother may have to listen to hours, sometimes days, of conflicting submissions and evidence about her capacity to care adequately for her children. Much of what she hears is likely to make her feel adversarial herself; but she will be no match for any of the solicitors who question her. Her accent and her colloquialisms may all be met with strained brows, looks of incredulity. She may often be asked to repeat herself and can easily be made to feel a fool. She may experience a powerful urge to cry out in anger or frustration, but her instincts are likely to tell her that courtrooms are seldom sympathetic to feelings, no matter how justified. At the end of the proceedings, she may walk away devastated, her conviction in her own caring capacities shattered. Her solicitor may commiserate with her, but he is unlikely to accompany her; ironically, her only support at that point in time may be the social worker who has played a central role in the court's decision that her children remain in care.

Lack of preparation

As with case conference participation, considerable efforts are made to prepare childcare professionals, particularly social workers, for care proceedings, and little if any effort is made to prepare mothers. Childcare professionals demand training for court, even before they qualify. They are acutely aware of the challenges in court. King and Trowell (1992) remark:

'It is disturbing when social workers seem more anxious about court procedures, legal strategies, rules of evidence, and how to give a good performance in court than about child development and the most effective way of helping' (p. 7). It is mothers more than anyone else who need preparation. They are usually less confident, less articulate, and less educated. For them, the stakes are highest; the atmosphere, ritual and formality, are strange and threatening; the language often jargonistic and incomprehensible; and, the prospect of walking to the witness stand, terrifying. (Some of the locations in which witnesses have to give evidence are indeed daunting even for hardened professionals; the author recalls a court in which no witness stand existed; each witness had to give evidence standing in a large space of floor before the clerk and magistrates.)

Comprehensive assessment

The Department of Health's (1988) publication on comprehensive assessment *Protecting Children* is widely used throughout childcare agencies. The timing of its publication was significant, shortly after public enquiry reports on ill-treatment, neglect, and murders of children (Blom-Cooper 1985; Greenwich 1987; Lambeth 1987), and just before publication of numerous, voluminous regulations and guides on the Children Act 1989. The assessment guide is the culmination of the Government's attempts throughout the 1980s to impose increasingly detailed regulation and procedure upon childcare workers. The aim was to minimize risk by maximizing authority in and control of allegedly abusive situations. McBeath and Webb (1990–1) made a detailed study of the guide and underlined its distinctly authoritative tone and stance. Two potentially abusive features of the Department of Health guide are immediately apparent. First, it is so comprehensive and all-embracing that many of the hundreds of questions it contains are intrusive, repetitive or irrelevant (O'Hagan 1993), and to be frank, no parent, let alone any single unsupported mother, needs to be or deserves to be subjected to so many questions. On too few occasions, the authors limply recommend some discretion; on too many occasions they stress thoroughness and completion. All questions are given equal prominence in the way they are listed. Clearly, the authors do not subscribe to the common sense of Coulshed (1991) who writes: 'the skill in doing assessment ... lies in an ability to collect enough, but not too much information' (p. 27). Second, as in the Children Act, the guide consistently refers to 'parents', meaning the natural parents of the child. Partners of parents may be included in the assessment 'depending on the circumstances' (DoH 1988: 21). The reality in practice, as every child protection worker knows, is that many natural fathers have long disappeared from the scene and have been replaced by substitute father figures, who are transient, with no knowledge of or commitment to the child in question, and unwilling to be subjected to the scrutiny of an assessment. Consequently, mothers are the primary focus of the guide, the only person capable of answering the countless questions they will be asked. In addition to these two obvious features, there is another serious flaw in the guide: nowhere is there any awareness of the crisis nature of much childcare work. We will consider that in the light of another case.

> Josephine is an Afro-Caribbean mother of three children, aged seven, four and two. Her main income is provided by prostitution in an inner city. She returned home one night and found her children had been removed into care; an anonymous referral had alerted the authorities to the fact that the children were alone. Workers visited, spoke to neighbours, and tried to find Josephine, without success. They then decided to remove the children on emergency child protection orders. When Josephine finds out, she is devastated and cannot control her anger. She is not told of the children's whereabouts on that first night. She has to wait until the morning before seeing the relevant workers. They interview her, insofar as her anger will permit. She swears that the children were not supposed to be alone; that her childminders did not turn up at the appointed time, that she was convinced they would turn up, and that she was only leaving her children for 15 minutes.
>
> She is allowed contact with the children, but social services decide to: (1) keep them in emergency fostering accommodation; (2) hold a case conference (which Josephine is permitted to attend, though is excluded during the discussion and decision making); and (3) pursue care orders. In the court, much is made of the facts that Josephine works in prostitution, that her children have different fathers, and that numerous referrals have been made by her neighbours alleging neglect of the children. Her lawyer is able to confirm that none of these have ever been substantiated, and that the general health of the children is good. Nevertheless, care orders are obtained, and Josephine is informed that her children will remain in the foster home and that she will be permitted frequent contact. She is told that a 'comprehensive assessment' has now to be made.
>
> Throughout the following weeks a number of professionals are introduced to Josephine. Their combined perceptions of her are primarily negative – they find her angry, unforgiving, obstructive, contemptuous, despairing, suicidal, morose and indifferent. Some realize that it is pointless provoking her with questions about her 'early childhood and subsequent history and background'; about her 'personality and attitudes'; or about the origins and character of the fathers of her children. Unfortunately some do not realize, and when one worker asks her how she would describe herself in '*appearance, personality, and her feelings about herself*', she tells him to 'f—— off!'

This is the type of scenario much beloved by those dramatists who wish to caricature childcare workers, but regrettably, it is also fact. Cooper (1993) reminds us how enthusiastically childcare workers embrace the all-encompassing checklist types of diagnostic and assessment tools, as though they were indeed the 'maintenance mechanics' Davies (1991) claimed social workers to be. Such a role and such enthusiasm for playing it are seen to be disastrous in the above case. The fundamental mistake is in not realizing the impact upon Josephine of the initial intervention and removal; it has in effect profoundly undermined her emotional and psychological condition, and her social status. To expect her to respond positively to any attempt at assessment is naive in the extreme. Her experience of the intervention is such that she will behave in a way which succeeds only in confirming the view that she is an unfit and unreasonable mother.

There is not the slightest awareness in the DoH guide of the crisis nature of child protection work. There is, as has already been acknowledged, a helpful distinction made between investigation/intervention (when the crisis is generated) and, assessment. But there is no appreciation of the extent of the differences between the investigative/intervention phase, and the assessment phase, in terms of the feelings of the protagonists, the challenge to the workers, and the atmosphere in which they work. The guide says nothing about the probability that any mother from whom children have been removed (in her eyes unjustly), is unlikely to be able to cooperate, freely, genuinely and willingly, for the purposes of a comprehensive assessment. It says nothing about the paramount need of the workers to first bring about the necessary changes in the conflictual atmosphere and relationships between the mother and the principal intervening agencies. Social work literature and training have been neglectful of conflict in childcare practice (O'Hagan 1984, 1986, 1991) and perhaps it is unrealistic to expect a government publication to do otherwise. But any professional who reads Josephine's case must realize that the crisis and conflict which the investigation and intervention have caused, have to be faced; ignoring or forgetting the crisis and conflict ensures the worst possible prospect – an abusive prospect – for the comprehensive assessment which follows.

Fostering

When the decision to foster a child is made, professionals will rightly be preoccupied with the child's welfare, and they will make every effort to ensure that the foster parents have all the support and material means to facilitate a successful placement. These preoccupations often exclude the rights and needs of the parents of the child, despite the attention given to parental rights and responsibilities in the Children Act. The 'parents' caught up in fostering situations in which their children are placed are predominantly single parent mothers. Natural fathers have often long disappeared from the scene, and the substitute father figures who often temporarily replace them are usually extremely unwilling to get involved with foster parents. It is mothers, therefore, who often stand alone during the fostering phase.

Although the preoccupation with the welfare of the child is paramount during this (and every other) phase of childcare work, it is often the case that the welfare of the child in a fostering situation is inextricably dependent upon the degree of sensitivity and empathy professionals and foster parents demonstrate to the mother. Unfortunately for the child, sensitivity and empathy are often lacking; worse still, the fostering phase may be the one in which mothers first experience blatant abuse and hostility.

Mothers are abused in the fostering phase whenever:

1 they are not informed of the identity or the address of the foster parents;
2 they are prevented from having contact with the foster parents;
3 the child is moved from one foster parent to another without the mother knowing;
4 the child is placed so far away that the mother is discouraged from making the journey;
5 the mother is being assessed by professionals while she is visiting her child in the foster home;
6 the foster parents are given responsibility for investigating whether or not the mother has abused her child, or, given primary responsibility for assessing the mother's parenting capacities while she visits her child in the foster home;
7 the mother's request for her child to be brought up in accordance with certain racial, religious, or cultural norms, is ignored.

Those who believe that such abuses are highly unlikely may justifiably point to current childcare laws and policies, some of which may appear expressly to forbid them. But as always, childcare managers may exercise much discretion, and if they so judge these basic rights to be 'not in the child's best interests', they have the authority to deny them. There is also the issue of resources; there simply may not be suitable foster parents near enough to the child's home; social workers may not have the time to accompany and transport mothers too far away from placements (for example, one mother interviewed in O'Hagan's (1994b) research said the social worker never once succeeded in getting her to the foster home in time, and never once failed to collect her at the time she was due to leave!). The shortage of fostering resources may also be a contributory factor to the abuse of women. Because of this shortage, local authorities are compelled to accept foster parents who stipulate that they *do not* come into contact with the mother (for example, the authors recall attending a case conference in which the foster parents were 'smuggled' into and out of the conference through the back of the building, to avoid any contact with the single parent mother waiting at the front of the building). Some managers and frontline workers see nothing wrong with this stipulation; it is in fact, deeply insulting to any mother, and more importantly, it is an almost certain guarantee that the fostering and any proposed rehabilitation of the child back with the mother, will fail.

Most children aged between 2 and 12, being fostered, remain steadfastly loyal to their mother, no matter what abuse the mother may have inflicted upon them. It is crucially important for children to know that the world at large and significant people in that world, such as foster parents and professionals with whom they are often in contact, value and respect their mother as much as they (the children) do themselves. Children are remarkably acute in sensing foster parents' criticism or resentment of their mother (foster parents deceive themselves if they believe it is okay to be critical of parents provided the child does not hear you criticize them; foster parents' criticism and resentment of mothers will manifest itself in numerous ways besides the spoken word, and children will sense it). The fostered children will often be deeply hurt and angered on learning or sensing that the foster parents do not like their mother. Younger children are unlikely to be able to verbalize these feelings, either to the foster parents or the visiting professionals. But such feelings will be expressed none the less, either through withdrawal and apathy, or through self-destructiveness or aggression. Very often, these feelings will be expressed when the child has been returned to the foster home, having had contact with the mother; ironically, the foster parents will see the mother as the cause of the child's distress and/or acting out, a perception which may, tragically, be shared by the professionals.

Race, religion, culture

Considering point 7 in the above list, the Children Act and the subsequent policy and procedural statements based upon it emphasize the right of parents to request that their child be brought up in a particular faith and culture, and that it is the duty of professionals to ensure that such a request is granted. But there are so many other necessary and complex tasks in fostering, that workers and their managers can easily regard this duty as less important than the law, policy and procedure make out. Mothers lacking confidence and assertiveness are unlikely to insist upon this right; consequently, their sense of identity and the relationship with their child, both evolving within a religious and/or cultural context, can be undermined when such a right is ignored. In contrast, localities and agencies in which there are prevailing and politically significant cultural, ethnic or religious characteristics, are likely to ensure no deviation from the policy.

For example, no professional could ignore the above request made by a black Afro-Caribbean mother in a locality predominantly inhabited by Afro-Caribbean people, with a flourishing Afro-Caribbean culture. Similarly, no professional in Belfast could remove a child from the Protestant Shankill Road and ignore the mother's request by placing the child in the Catholic Falls Road. The fact is, however, that there are many fostering situations in which no such culture and its inevitable pressures exist. Mothers' requests for their children to be placed with foster parents of the same religion as that in which the child was brought up, are very often ignored or quickly forgotten in many parts of the UK. This may stem from a predominantly secular, humanist ethos among childcare staff.

Case history

Another form of abuse of mothers during the fostering phase occurs when foster parents, rather than avoiding natural mothers, become over involved in the process of assessment. This is best illustrated through a case history.

> Barbara is a 23 year old single parent mother whose child Paul, aged 3, was removed on the grounds of neglect and failure-to-thrive. He was placed with Mr and Mrs Matthews. Social services intend carrying out a comprehensive assessment, in which the views of the Matthews, particularly Mrs Matthews, will be crucial.
>
> Barbara is regarded as a difficult client, volatile and unreliable. She has had a history characterized by deprivation, special education, care and abuse. She resents authority of any kind. She is deeply resentful of her child's removal and placement with a foster parent. She detests visiting the foster home, but social services have told her contact with her child will only take place in the foster home.
>
> Barbara is being assessed through interviews with numerous professionals, and by being observed in interaction with her child during contact in the foster home. Mrs Matthews, a very experienced foster parent, is asked to make these observations and record them for social services.
>
> Barbara is invariably tense when visiting the foster home. She knows she is being watched and assessed by the woman who is caring for her son. No matter how friendly Mrs Matthews is, Barbara cannot relax, cannot be friendly in return. She is acutely conscious of the material wealth in the home, the fact that Paul is surrounded by colourful and expensive educational toys, that he wears clothes which she cannot afford to buy for him.

It is quite common for mothers to be 'assessed' for their parenting capacities in an environment in which it will be difficult for them to demonstrate any such capacities. It is not uncommon for the foster mother, often the object of extreme resentment, fear and envy on the part of the natural mother (particularly when no preparatory work has been done in establishing a working, mutually respectful relationship between the two), to be given the onerous task of recording and reporting her observations of the interactions between mother and child in this wholly inappropriate environment. The imbalance of power in this assessment equation, and the abuse which it constitutes, can be magnified further when all the professionals involved increasingly rely upon the foster mother's views, and increasingly avoid contact with the mother. It is infinitely less challenging and thoroughly more pleasant working with nice middle-class foster parents than attempting to work with young, damaged and volatile single parent mothers.

Adoption

Adoption will often be the final phase in childcare work for all the parties concerned. For the mother of the child, it is likely to be the most difficult and traumatic phase. Mothers in Howe *et al.* (1992) speak of being 'totally negated as people throughout the Adoption process' (p. 128). There is a plethora of research and literature on the subjects of 'the adopted child' and on the 'prospective parents', and on the needs of both; in contrast, there is very little research and literature available on the experiences and needs of the birth mothers.

The abuse of women during the adoption phase may first be seen within a global dimension: the number of children available for adoption in Western countries, and, the number of adoption orders, have drastically fallen in recent years. 'Healthy babies are a scarce commodity' says Thoburn (1993: 1). Prospective adopters however, have had their prospects of adopting a child greatly enhanced by wars and revolutions in various parts of the world (for example, Romania, the former Yugoslavia, etc.); Thoburn warns of the exploitation, abuses and corruption which may stem from such cases; press and television have provided countless examples of the same. It is invariably the mothers of the adopted children, who are the victims of this abuse and corruption.

The origins of the abuse of women in adoption lie in social, political and legal history. We have learnt that Houghton's (1972) idealistic notion of partnership between mothers and adoption agencies and the introduction of freeing orders to promote the same, have actually led to a dramatic increase in the number of contested adoptions (Lambert *et al.* 1989; Lowe 1993; see also Chapter 5, this volume). We have learnt from parents themselves about some of the conflictual consequences (Howe *et al.* 1992; Hendry and Scourfield 1994). Now we can identify precisely the principal women-abusive features of the whole adoption process.

They may be classified under attitude/perception and action: first, negative and/or patriarchal perceptions of mothers whose children are born out of wedlock. There is a prevailing 'negativeness' in the perceptions of single parent mothers today, cultivated and supported by blatantly hostile pronouncements of government ministers, and right-wing ideological treatises on the menace of an increasing population of single parent mothers. This negativeness constitutes an additional pressure upon those mothers contemplating whether or not to keep their children. Patriarchal-type perceptions may be more sympathy based, but they are no less unhelpful for that. The mothers involved may be perceived as unfortunate, deprived, poverty stricken, misled, young girls, who have to be taken care of by male-managed childcare agencies, and male-dominated judicial processes. This type of 'taking-care-of' perceives adoption as the solution to the increasing 'one parent family problem'. It takes little account of the innermost feelings of mothers and is incapable of foreseeing the long-term consequences of adoption upon the mother. Worse, it does not even credit mothers with the capacity to change from the original damaging perception in which they are held; they are for ever perceived as immature and irresponsible. This has serious consequences for those mothers who apply to have the right of contact with their adopted children, by virtue of the Children Act 1989 (s. 8). This right is already a subject of much controversy and uncertainty (Lowe 1993; Triseliotis 1993). Lowe's opinion is that 'only in exceptional circumstances' will birth mothers be permitted to apply for a Section 8 contact order. Hendry and Scourfield (1994) predict a two-tier system of adoption, that is, a court's response to the request for information and contact will depend upon whether or not the birth mother has consented to the adoption.

Second, in the light of the evidence (Lambert *et al.* 1989; Howe *et al.* 1992; Lowe 1993), applications for freeing orders do create conflict. There is enormous imbalance between the two sides in the conflict, that is, powerful established agencies with their highly experienced legal representatives, and single mothers, often unsupported, often disowned by their families of origin, and often recovering from the trauma of births which many people tried to persuade them not to have. Single mothers are likely to lose in this conflict. There is some evidence in Lowe (1993) to suggest that freeing applications are actually used to control and direct the conflict: 'Agencies feel that the advantages of freeing in such cases is that it protects the prospective adopters by alleviating some of their anxiety because it is the adoption agency which takes on the contest with the natural parents' (p. 13). Lowe (1993) suggests that earlier research (Triseliotis and Hall 1971) raises serious questions about the usefulness of conflict laden freeing orders; they were introduced to deal with and put an end to mothers repeatedly changing their mind about adoption. But Triseliotis and Hall demonstrate that the period of most frequent change of mind is *during the first six weeks following the birth,* a time when no formal decision or agreement can be made in any case. There is no research evidence indicating that mothers continue to change their minds after that six week period.

Third, the economic, social and personal pressures on pregnant women to give up their child to adoption, have been well documented (for example, Shawyer 1979; Reich 1988; Howe *et al.* 1992). Childcare agencies to whom these women are directed, and with whom they will inevitably come into contact, may add to the pressures by not providing the necessary resources enabling them to surmount whatever social and economic difficulties they encounter.

Fourth, mothers who decide before the birth to place their child for adoption may be persuaded that it would be best for the child to be removed at birth and that it is not in their interests to see the child. This used to be a common practice necessitating the cooperation of medical and nursing services.

Fifth, in response to the initial trauma of separation, mothers may be told that they have done the right thing both for their child and for themselves and that the pain will eventually ease: 'you will learn to live with it'. They seldom do and are likely to endure self-doubt as a consequence: 'there must be something wrong with me if I am not able to live with it as suggested'.

Sixth, the attempts to persuade mothers to 'learn to live with it' are at variance to some extent with the increasing rights of adopted children to trace and make contact with their natural parents. Mothers have little control over these processes, whether they desire to see their adult child or not and irrespective of their current situation and relationships. Howe *et al.*'s (1992) study documents the joy and ecstacy experienced by some mothers, but also, the terror and devastation felt by others, when their adult children succeed in tracing them.

Seventh, there is no lasting post-adoption service for the vast majority of mothers who give up their child to adoption. Consequently, the pain and trauma arising from many of the above abuses intensifies, and seldom disappears.

Finally, in many adoptions, particularly those which follow the compulsory removal of children against the wishes of the mother, mothers may be denied any information about the child's welfare and progress. For all mothers in all adoption cases this lack of information can be a source of much anguish (Hendry and Scourfield 1994). They naturally have prolonged periods of wondering and worrying about how their children are doing, or hoping and praying they are doing well. Yet they can be reluctant and too frightened to make contact with agencies which have forgotten about them. Mothers speak of the enormous psychological difficulty in doing so, and of the cold, suspicious reactions they often get from new staff in those agencies who raise questions about their motivation (Howe *et al.* 1992). Mothers of black children who have been adopted speak of their fears of their children suffering from racism, or, whether or not their black heritage 'was being acknowledged or valued, or denied' (Howe *et al.* 1992: 129). Often mothers will experience powerful impulses to seek out their child and find out for themselves. One mother recorded:

I kept asking the social services department for news of Vicki and Sarah but they kept telling me I wasn't allowed any because my access had been stopped and my children had been adopted anyway. They just seemed to think I could go away and forget all about them. (Hendry and Scourfield 1994: 28)

Conclusion

This chapter has demonstrated the profound and pervasive nature of the abuse of women throughout all phases of child protection and childcare work. It has done so chiefly through the use of case material – that is, actual examples of the abuse of women. Considerable time has been given to the abuse of women during the initial *referral* phase. This is a phase often neglected in training. Consequently, professionals and managers have not had the opportunity to learn of the complexities and the challenges which various categories of referrals present (particularly anonymous referrals), and of the risk of laying the foundations of women-abusive attitudes and actions at such an early stage. In *investigation*, professionals may focus on mothers despite allegations that the abuser was her male partner; they may allow alarming or damning file reports of the past to establish unshakeable perceptions of the present, even before they visit the mother; they may attempt to see and question the child without a mother knowing, and they may be less than honest with both parent and child at various stages of their investigation.

There are many potential abuses during the *intervention* phase, particularly revolving around medical examinations. Additionally, workers may intervene without having made any assessment of the general welfare of the child – that is, the emotional, psychological, social and educational life of the child, all of which may indicate a high quality of care provided by mothers. Mothers are often abused during the *case conference* phase; ironically, the right to attend case conferences has proved to be even more abusive for some mothers than the right not to attend; this is mainly due to the lack of preparation of parents. Policy and procedure on the convening of case conferences are often too crudely all-embracing; the whole paraphernalia of case conference may be inflicted upon mothers without any justification. Mothers often endure great hardship and trauma during *care proceedings*. As in the case conference phase, they are are totally ill-prepared for many aspects of the courtroom experience, particularly the adversarial nature of proceedings, and the anxiety-laden challenge they face in being questioned by so many solicitors. *Comprehensive assessment* is a crucially important phase in childcare work. But the model provided by DoH (1988) has proved to be intrusive, repetitive and irrelevant when its multiple checklists have been applied without discretion. More importantly, professionals have not always been aware that many mothers are traumatized by events in previous phases and are unable to cooperate for the purpose of assessment. Mothers may be abused in numerous ways during the *fostering* phase. They may be denied contact with the foster parent; their children's perceptions of them may be undermined or manipulated by foster parents' hostility or indifference; the mother's requests and/or stipulations about race, culture, or religion may be forgotten or ignored; the foster parents may be over-involved in the assessment of the mother; assessment of the mother's parenting capacities may be carried out through observing her, and her interactions with her child, in the home of the foster parents. Finally, the testimony of mothers and the available research has amply demonstrated that the *adoption* phase, world-wide, is a minefield of abusive procedures and practices, originating primarily from potentially abusive legislation.

9

The abuse of women by avoiding men

Introduction

The abuse of women takes many forms. One of the most common is the avoidance of men. A number of questions arise: first, what is meant by the avoidance of men, and how can that be construed as (or how might it lead to) the abuse of women? Second, what, if any, is the relationship between the avoidance of men and, the theoretical and practical exploration of the abuse of women made in previous chapters? This chapter will begin with a working definition of avoidance, followed by an explanation of how each of the various ways of avoiding men can easily lead to the abuse of women. There is undoubtedly a relationship between the avoidance of men and developmental theories which compel professionals to concentrate upon women; and there are specific features of abusive childcare systems conducive to the avoidance of men. But another reason why childcare professionals avoid men is less complex: it is fear of violence and intimidation. Numerous examples of this type of avoidance will be provided from child abuse enquiry reports, including the testimony of workers involved. The chapter will demonstrate how fear of men perceived as violent can easily lead to different types of abuse of women and abusive consequences for the child.

Definition of 'avoidance'

Avoiding people usually means taking some action which ensures you do not come into contact with them. Avoiding men in childcare work means something more. First, it can mean that the context in which one works – that is, its structure and organization, its demands and preoccupations –

makes it extremely difficult for the worker *not* to avoid men. Milner is an academic highly conscious of this matter; yet when she returned to childcare practice for a short period, she later asked herself:

> How is it that a system which I experienced as oppressively scrutinis-ing, permitted me to shift from the main aim of investigation: bringing forward potentially dangerous fathers and/or highlighting dangerous situations? That I managed largely to ignore fathers is even more surprising when I consider the knowledge base which informed my practice. (1993: 49)

The word 'ignore' is later upgraded to 'avoid', as the writer admits some culpability within the women-abusive context she is describing: 'Whilst I was consciously aware that I was conspiring with a system which scrutinised mothering, I was not as aware of my complicity in a process which avoids scrutinising fathering' (p. 59).

Second, avoidance may mean making no effort to understand either the significance of men in childcare, particularly child abuse situations, or the relationship which men have with the mothers of children allegedly abused. Third, it more commonly means avoiding not just the contact and scrutiny to which Milner refers, but also, more importantly, avoiding the challenging and necessary interactions with men, and the absence of honesty and frankness in one's professional contact with them.

Many of the child abuse enquiry reports provide examples of these types of avoidance. The social workers and health visitors in the case of Kimberly Carlile (Greenwich 1987) avoided Mr Carlile at any cost; they did have contact with Nigel Hall, the man who eventually murdered Kimberly, but the quality of that contact was such that it did nothing to protect her, and may have been a contributory factor in the abuse and death which she suffered. The social worker and health visitor in the Jasmine Beckford (Blom-Cooper 1985) case had numerous contacts with Morris Beckford (78 recorded visits to the home). But the relationship they established with him was based upon a degree of naivety on their part which precluded them even attempting to understand him, either his relationship with Jasmine's mother, or his potential for violence towards mother and child alike. Andrew Neil, the murderer of Tyra Henry (Lambeth 1987) provoked the same blatant avoidance tactics as those in the Carlile case. It is one report which examines this avoidance and its consequences in some depth. In contrast, there was little comment on the professionals' avoidance of Frank Kepple, the man who killed Maria Colwell (DHSS 1974). The social worker took over the case in April 1970, but, says the report nonchalantly: 'She was not able to meet Mr Kepple until November, and then only very briefly on the steps of a public house' (p. 16).

When does avoidance occur?

The avoidance of men may occur during any one of the phases of childcare work. One may automatically assume that it occurs more frequently during the investigation or intervention phase, but as the previous chapter demonstrated, its roots may well be established in the attitudes and actions of professionals during the initial referral phase.

Avoidance during the referral phase

Avoidance of men occurs during the referral phase when those taking the referral concentrate their questioning on mothers, and ask few if any questions about male partners. The avoidance of men is intensified if the questioning tends to identify the mother as the one responsible for the abuse (no need to bother about the man in that case). This is the most common form of avoidance during the referral phase, and most probably will influence the investigation which follows. A less obvious kind of avoidance – indeed, one which appears to be the very opposite to avoidance – occurs when the referrer actually does ask many questions about the male partner; however, these questions focus primarily on any perceived dangerousness in the partner. From the relative safety of the duty office, the professional may ask about the man's criminal past, his violent tendencies, his hostility to childcare workers, etc. The principal reason for these questions is to alert the investigating officer about how difficult this man may be, thus clearly implying that he should be avoided.

Avoiding men during the investigative phase

There are basically two forms of avoidance of men during investigation. First, as we have seen often in previous chapters, workers may ensure that they make their investigative visit at a time when the man will not be present. Second, workers can just as easily avoid meaningful, necessary and challenging contact with men who are present. This is a more dangerous form of avoidance, yet very common in practice, and much in evidence in the cases of Beckford (Blom-Cooper 1985), Carlile (Greenwich 1987), and Sukina (Bridge 1991). This avoidance occurs when questions are addressed solely to the woman. The man sits there, listening, or not listening, reading his newspaper, or watching the 2.30 at Newmarket, relieved in sensing that he is not going to be asked anything. This type of avoidance is more common if the man is not known or is a new boyfriend or cohabitee. This provides the excuse that it would be an infringement on his liberty to ask him any questions, when the real reason is simply a lack of confidence on the part of the worker. Holding back from what one wants to say because the man is present is another form of avoidance. The workers may talk about peripheral matters in the hope that the man will eventually leave. This is more difficult and dangerous for both worker and mother.

Avoiding men during the intervention phase

Men may be avoided during the intervention phase by any of the following means:

1 They are not invited to attend medical examinations, or, medicals are arranged at a time when men cannot attend. There are occasions when professionals believe a suspected man's presence at a medical examination is detrimental to the investigation and not in the child's interests; this may be the case, but, more often than not, the reason why men do not attend medicals is because professionals have not encouraged them to attend, nor facilitated them attending.
2 Child protection orders may be invoked without reference to a male partner present in the home, or, a male partner significant to the child.
3 In cases of neglect and/or abandonment, rigorous searches are invariably made for the mother, despite the husband/partner's equal responsibility.
4 Mothers are likely to be the principal focus of any caution or warning to parents; male partners may not be seen.
5 In cases of child sexual abuse in particular, suspected potential abusers are avoided, and pressure is put on mothers to get them removed.
6 Preparations for case conferences will focus upon the mother; the workers may ignore the male partner, whatever his significance.

Avoiding men during the case conference phase

All the various types of avoidances of men during both the investigation and intervention phases will be mirrored in official recordings and reports necessary during these phases – that is, case recordings, case conference reports, court reports, etc. The avoidances are likely to have originated in referral taking. Case conference and court reports are notoriously lacking of information about male partners (O'Hagan 1989, 1993). In the case of Sukina (Bridge 1991), there were eight case conferences over a period of three years, attended by no less than 54 professionals; yet there was no crucial information available in the literally hundreds of reports provided by these professionals, about the character and personality of the father who brutally murdered her because she could not spell her name. Common utterances at case conferences attended by the authors over many years, include: 'what's this new partner like ... I haven't had the chance to meet him ... there's some new bloke living with her now ... what do we know about this character? ... he never has much to say for himself', etc. Parental attendance at case conferences may improve the situation, but research clearly indicates the predictable tendency of mothers attending conferences alone (O'Hagan 1994b). Professionals find it difficult enough adjusting to the presence of mothers; they will be in no hurry to encourage fathers to attend case conferences, and they will be quite capable of discouraging them from doing so.

Avoiding men in care proceedings

Court proceedings and court reports often reveal the avoidance of men. Magistrates and judges are not likely (even with the Children Act) to kick up a fuss when men are absent, or when court reports say little or nothing about male partners. Thus no one protested at the absence of Frank Kepple, the killer of Maria Colwell (DHSS 1974) during crucial care proceedings in November 1971. It was left to Mrs Kepple to answer the key question 'what was Mr Kepple's attitude to Maria?' to which she replied: 'he treats Maria as one of his own children' (p. 30).

Avoiding men during the fostering phase

In many fostering cases, the avoidance of men will be blatant; foster parents will simply demand that they have no contact with the child's parents, particularly a father/male partner who is the alleged or proven abuser. Childcare workers will be compelled to comply with this demand and, indeed, may welcome it. Where foster parents are less demanding, they and workers may still place obstacles in the way of contact with male partners. Arrangements for parent(s)–child contact, may only facilitate *mother–child* contact. Convictions for violence or records of hostility towards professionals may be greatly emphasized to foster parents, indeed, may be projected by the worker onto the foster parents, with the hope that the foster parents will see the male partner precisely as the worker sees him.

Avoiding men in long-term assessment and rehabilitation

Childcare professionals have traditionally avoided men and concentrated upon women in assessment and rehabilitation work. Women are analysed, counselled, taught (for example, childcare skills, domestic management, assertiveness, etc.), encouraged or persuaded to attend family centres, playgroups, nursery school, etc., all for the purpose of increasing their child-rearing capabilities and enhancing the quality of their relationship with their children.

Corresponding with these efforts is an obvious tendency to avoid any similar work with her male partner, based upon an equally obvious lack of awareness about the influence (good or bad) which the male partner may have upon the results of their efforts. Probably the best known example of this type of avoidance phenomenon in long-term work with a mother is in Dale *et al.* (1986). The work has been criticized (Hearn 1990; Parton 1990) for its patriarchal stance in which mainly male workers impose a rigidly controlled programme upon a young mother, 'Sandra', apparently with some success. More interesting, however, is the worker's attitude to her boyfriend, David, the father of the child. As noted above, various types of avoidances of David are already in play; for example, we are provided with much information about the character, personality and background of Sandra (including a psychiatric history), but virtually none at all about David. David proves to be something of an obstacle to all these male workers attempting to help Sandra; so, in an extraordinary and very revealing phrase, the authors write: 'He was defined out with Sandra's agreement' (Dale *et al.*: 136). This may be convenient, but it is not intelligent, as subsequent reading indicates; we hear nothing more about David, except, after the 'successful' rehabilitation: 'It has not been possible to describe the complex relationship between Sandra and her boyfriend . . . she continued to express ambivalent and contradictory feelings of wanting both proximity and distance from him' (p. 149). This makes it inexplicable why, other than the conscious or unconscious need to avoid him, the workers did not persist in including the father in their attempt at rehabilitation.

Explanation: how is avoidance of men abusive to women?

The abusive consequences of blatant avoidance

There are as many answers to this question as there are types of avoidance, and we can begin by looking at the avoidance demonstrated in Chapter 1, and in a number of cases in the previous chapter. That very common type of blatant avoidance – that is, ensuring that the man is not present during the investigative visit – can have numerous effects. First, it renders the woman alone to face two educated, articulate and determined professionals (often police and social worker combined), who will inflict a major crisis upon her. The imbalance of power in this situation is gross, and the woman's anxiety, fear and vulnerability will be acute.

Second, her ability to function as an adequate mother is jeopardized by these kind of unannounced investigative visits. No worker can fail to notice the dramatic change in the woman's demeanour – her mood, her eyes, her voice, etc. – on hearing of the purpose of the visit. More importantly, the investigation can instantly transform the interactions and relationships between the woman and her children from that of normality, to that of mutual incredulity, fear, even terror (see investigative phase in previous chapter, in the case of 'Maureen'. Also, the author can recall numerous investigative visits in which mothers ran terrified from one room to another, leaving their equally terrified children in the presence of stranger social workers). Women may realize the impact of the visit upon their interactions with their children, but may be helpless in doing anything about it. They may realize too the impact upon their children and be acutely aware that they are incapable of rescuing and comforting the children throughout the duration of the visit. One of the worst forms of the abuse of women may then follow: the investigative workers record in their files how insensitive this mother was to her children. They may, for example, write something like this: 'during our initial and follow up visits, the children were very distressed and *she ignored them; she had no empathy with them; she was preoccupied with herself and what may happen to her as a consequence of our visit*'.

Third, the mother is left to explain the investigative visit when the man returns. The difficulty and risk in this task will be determined by the character and perceptions of the male partner, and whether or not he is the abuser (he often is, which makes the visit to the lone mother unfair and ironical). He may be indifferent, shocked, angry, baffled or scared; he may be a volatile, aggressive type of person, or extremely suspicious, or imbued with an all-consuming fear and hatred of police and/or childcare workers. He may choose the pub as the quickest and most certain remedy to the news, and re-enter the scene paralytic, cursing and fuming about diabolical health visitors and social workers and what he will do to them, etc. (Nigel Hall, in the Carlile case (Greenwich 1987) reacted to the news of social work enquiries by making a dramatic, unannounced, appearance in the reception hall of the local office: 'he appeared angry and edgy, even aggressive ... almost shouting: "social workers: the worst people who walk the earth"' (p. 68)). This is not the kind of behaviour that the woman needs in her moment of crisis. On the other hand, her partner may choose to stay well clear of the professionals; he may reciprocate their own behaviour by focusing upon her; he may interrogate her, trying to find out if she has said something she should not have said; dreading that they have won her over to their side, and that she is now colluding with them, betraying him. If he is a suspicious man, he may interpret his partner's crisis state – that is, her fear and panic – as proof of her guilt. If he is a violent man, he may attack her. It is sometimes difficult for middle-class, reasonable-minded professionals to imagine such consequences, but they do in fact occur frequently, and are often the logical consequence of the decision to visit the woman and avoid the man. Many of the child abuse enquiry reports reveal the climate of fear existing in the relationship between the victims' mothers and their male partners, and of the women's attempts to ensure they never did anything contrary to the wishes of the men. Investigating childcare professionals never intend that a woman may suffer interrogation and attack by her male partner as a consequence of their visit; regrettably, they are seldom aware that in some cases, such attack will be inevitable. Childcare professionals are never in control of the consequences of their investigative visit to a lone mother.

Abusive consequences of avoiding men who are present

Avoidance of men who are present can also be dangerously abusive to women. The banal conversation about peripheral matters (simply because the worker feels unable to be frank and honest in the man's presence) may actually provoke the man. Cryptic conversation, dependent upon tone and gesture, hoping at the same time that the man will eventually leave, may actually have the opposite effect of making him stay, making him suspicious of some kind of conspiracy and collusion between worker and mother. This is often a recipe for conflict in the relationship between man and woman when the worker departs, with adverse consequences for the welfare of the child. The authors recreate this professional dilemma in training sessions; students see the video recording of a role play, based upon a health visitor's predicament in this regard. She cannot ask about the bruising on the child because of the presence of the man, whom she suspects of perpetrating the abuse. The mother dangerously senses that the health visitor wants to talk to her about it. The health visitor refers the case to a child protection agency, and requests that she remain anonymous. What qualities, training, agency procedure, etc., would enable her to act differently?

Abusive consequences of avoiding men by 'defining them out'

Many professionals think of and act towards men as though men were unimportant and marginal to the childcare issue. Few childcare professionals try to engage men and fewer insist on men's involvement throughout any of the different phases of childcare work (how many paediatricians for example would insist on a father's presence during a medical examination?). This is particularly the case if the man is a boyfriend, or cohabitee, and not the natural father of the child. The consequence of all this avoidance is often a realization by the man that he *need not* get involved. If the case advances towards care proceedings, he will know that he will not be expected to appear on the witness stand and be interrogated by all those nasty lawyers. If the child is placed with foster parents, he knows that he is likely to be ignored; if the authorities decide on a comprehensive assessment, he will know that most if not all of the questions will not be addressed to him. In short, men quickly realize and mostly appreciate that they are being 'defined out' (Dale *et al.* 1986) of the whole childcare situation. The consequence for the mother is the realization that she really is alone; that it is she alone who will face the professionals throughout all phases of the case in question. This realization can make the mother feel more and more vulnerable as the case progresses through each phase.

Abusive consequences of avoiding men by 'trusting' mothers

Many childcare professionals are conscious of their tendencies to avoid men, particularly men known to be violent. Professionals may realize that there are certain dangers in this tendency, but they are unable to do anything about it. They compensate by making greater efforts in establishing relationships with the mother, supporting and encouraging the mother in good childcare practice, and, they hope, ensuring that she, the mother, will be able to protect the child from the violent male partner (O'Hagan 1989, 1993). Consequently, if things go wrong (as they often do given this naive, man-avoiding strategy), the mother will be held responsible: she did not protect her child (despite so many conversations about the danger, etc.); she must have colluded in the abuse of her child; she must have deceived the professionals who were doing everything to help her, etc.

What has actually happened in this case, is that professionals have attempted to invest in the mother a child-protective power and authority which they hope she will be able to exercise over her male partner. They have done this solely because they have failed to exercise their own very real power and authority over that same person. Most mothers will sense this; many will realize they are being given an impossible task: to protect their child from someone they themselves (and the professionals) have learnt to fear. Some will in the earlier stages have attempted to express their fear and doubt about this task: 'you don't know what he's like . . . I'm terrified of him . . . it doesn't make any difference what I say', etc., but there are no more dangerously effective balms than the reassuring reasonableness of childcare workers who would not want to be five minutes in the same room as the male partner, let alone having to live with him! The outcome is predictable: mothers will escape from this double bind either by accepting these naive reassurances, and, convincing themselves that all is well, or, they may begin deceiving the workers, concealing the fact that all is not well. This is the reason why, if something goes wrong, mothers are so severely criticized.

However, underlying these responses, the more fundamental reason is scapegoating: it is the professionals who have abused the mother and failed to protect the child primarily through their avoidance of the male partner; it is the mother who has to suffer most for their failings. The report into the death of Tyra Henry (Lambeth 1987) established that her killer Andrew Neil was as much avoided as he was feared; it then states:

It followed that Tyra was at risk from the moment she was conceived . . .
We cannot understand how those responsible for taking the ensuing

decisions can simultaneously have appreciated that Claudette [Tyra's mother] had probably not severed her links with Andrew, have recognised that she was in a difficult position, *and have then explicitly placed on her the entire responsibility for preparing to protect the second child from the man who had gravely injured the first, deferring any social services action until after the baby's birth.* (p. 20; emphasis added)

Abusive consequences of avoiding men by relying on grandmothers

When Tyra Henry was born, the childcare agencies unwittingly resorted to another very common abuse of women as a consequence of avoiding men. They regarded Andrew Neil as a serious risk, and Claudette Henry as a mother who would not be able to protect Tyra. They enlisted the support of Tyra's maternal grandparent to do the protecting for them. The report referred to the 'vice of the course decided on ... it accepted council responsibility for Tyra but sought to discharge it by delegating it wholesale to Beatrice Henry [Tyra's grandmother]'. Grandmothers can be made to feel important in this role, and can easily undermine the mother. The authors can recall many such cases from their own experiences. The mother is coerced into surrendering her child to the care of her own mother; there is the threat of a child protection order or care order if she does not. Thus the seeds of conflict are sown between the mother and grandparent, the mother compelled to live in circumstances increasingly humiliating, and understandably ready to reach out to anyone offering her an escape. Andrew Neil did so, and Claudette Henry's secret and not-so-secret rendezvous with him became more frequent (see Chapter 5, 'Grandmothers know best').

The reasons why childcare professionals avoid men

The reasons why childcare professionals avoid men are not precisely the same as the reasons why they concentrate on women. Some of the reasons for the avoidance are implicit and explicit in the two previous sections – that is, types of avoidance, and explanations on how avoidance constitutes an abuse of women. But there are sometimes more fundamental origins of the avoidance, origins which have been explored in previous chapters. For example, workers may genuinely believe that men are insignificant in the care and protection of children. That belief can be fostered in the workers' own personal experiences, in their observations of men in the homes of clients, and in what women clients actually tell them about their male partners, confirming more or less that it is the woman who is single-handedly caring for the child(ren). A more ideological stance may underpin the avoidance: men may be regarded as the principal source of all women's difficulties. This may also stem from personal experience, later consolidated in some feminist theory and literature. This can foster a hostile or contemptuous attitude towards men, a determination to avoid any contact or engagement with them, and subtle manipulation of the mother's feelings and perceptions of her male partner, attempting to enable her to leave. Men who repeatedly batter their female partners can make professionals even more determined to avoid having any contact with them. Many professionals quickly become aware in practice that they lack the skills, knowledge and confidence to engage men, particularly men with a reputation for violence. Childcare professionals commonly avoid men because of an anticipated violence and intimidation. This needs further exploration.

Violence against childcare workers

Childcare workers rightly believe their work is dangerous. Research and literature give some indication of the nature and extent of the problem (see for example, Rowett 1986; Norris 1991). One author worked for many years in a Divisional office which had 4 social work teams. There was at least one attack per month of varying degrees of severity on any one of the staff. One colleague was attacked by a male client wielding a knife and was seriously wounded. Another was attacked by a drunken male client, and was punched and kicked; another was attacked in a hospital waiting area by the father of a child being medically examined. Men have murdered social workers (Peter Gray, murdered in 1978; Francis Bettridge, in 1986). Violent men consistently dominate the 35 enquiry reports produced since 1974, and have, with very few exceptions, been responsible for the deaths of the children in those reports. Many of the mothers of these children were frequently battered by the men.

This knowledge, together with the chilling statistics on violence against childcare workers generally (including GPs and police involved in child protection work) fuel the anxiety of workers. Men who appear cold, arrogant, loud-mouthed, distant, resentful, or who are known women-batterers, or who have been convicted for offences of violence sometime in the past, are perceived as threatening and dangerous by many childcare workers. The paralysing effect of this perception, and the extent of effort in avoiding it, is indicated in a number of testimonies in the enquiry reports (though such feelings and avoidance are a daily occurrence in any childcare agency). A daycare member of staff in the case of Sukina (Bridge 1991), told the enquiry that she: 'dreaded being the senior person on duty if Sukina's father was going to collect her' (p. 86). The health visitor in the case of Kimberly Carlile (Greenwich 1987) described her feelings about visiting when Nigel Hall was home: 'the idea of visiting . . . was the sort of event that you would put off for a day when you are feeling particularly strong and able to cope with it' (p. 123).

The key worker involved in the case of Sudio Rouse (*The Observer* 1991) was apparently 'terrified' by the child's father, Robert Rouse, sentenced to life imprisonment for the murder of Sudio. Similar to the events in the Jasmine Beckford and Kimberly Carlile cases, the worker repeatedly visited and could not gain admission. Presumably this was an inconvenience more preferable than gaining admission and facing the men. The extent of avoidance of Andrew Neil, who killed his child Tyra Henry, seems proportionate to the preoccupation which many professionals shared about his potential for violence: there was so much discussion about him, in telephone calls, memos, letters and reports; so much concern, so many warnings . . . and yet, so much avoidance of him. The report comments: 'a major effort should have been made to involve Andrew Neil and his family constructively in plans for the child's welfare' (Lambeth 1987: 21).

Consequences of avoidance on the protection of children

It is obvious now how the avoidance of men can and often does constitute an abuse of women. But avoidance also seriously exacerbates the paramount task of protecting the child. In the opening paragraph of this chapter, one of the definitions of 'avoidance' was: 'avoiding challenging but necessary interactions with men'. These are crucial in child protection work. Without them (as we have seen in many of the case histories) the worker will be inhibited in asking the man legitimate questions about the child, the child's behaviour, marks or bruises on the child; the worker may be afraid to play and to communicate with the child in the man's presence, to disagree with assurances he gives; to express his/her own and other professionals' concerns, to suggest a doctor sees the child, to confront him directly and say he/she thinks he is trying to pull the wool over his/her eyes. There will be many occasions throughout the seven phases of childcare and child protection work when such interactions will be necessary. Anything less results in inadequacy in both assessment and protection. The protection of children cannot be achieved by the avoidance of men, whatever the reason may be for that avoidance. On the contrary, the increase in risk to a child in the same household may be directly proportionate to the extent to which professionals are attempting to avoid.

Conclusion

This chapter has demonstrated that the avoidance of men in childcare work is very common. Avoidance is manifest in various ways: ignoring men; making no attempt to engage them or understand their significance in the child abuse situation one may be investigating; or, more blatantly, visiting only when one is certain that men will not be present. Avoidance takes place throughout every phase of childcare work. Childcare workers are not always aware of their complicity in their agencies' avoidance of men generally (Milner 1993). Nor are they always aware of how avoidance may lead to the abuse of the woman partner. Each of the many differing types of abuses resulting from differing types of avoidance have been explored. Numerous reasons why childcare professionals avoid men, including reasons comprehensively explored in earlier chapters, have been suggested. One reason for avoidance is professionals' fear of intimidation and violence by men. Child abuse enquiry reports provide abundant evidence of how professionals may be influenced by fear of intimidation and violence. The inescapable conclusion is that the avoidance of men considerably increases the risk to the child.

PART III

The way ahead

10

Non-abusive childcare theory

Introduction

The potential for abuse in childcare systems has been widely recognized. In this book we have looked at some of the main causes and the most prevalent manifestations of this kind of abuse. The potential for abuse exists for any client who comes into contact with abusive childcare systems. We have focused on the abuse of women because women clients predominate in childcare. It is time to look for solutions and map out a way ahead which aims to prevent the abuse of women in childcare work and protect women as well as children.

In Part III we will look for an approach to childcare work which prevents the abuse of women. We will search for a framework which is designed to protect women and children in childcare work. We suggest that a major reappraisal and re-evaluation is necessary on a number of levels to ensure that the abuse described in this book no longer happens. The following three chapters will offer the beginnings of such a reappraisal or re-evaluation in relation to childcare theory (Chapter 10), childcare laws and procedures (Chapter 11), and the training of childcare workers (Chapter 12). Some of the thoughts and ideas described in these chapters will be familiar to childcare workers, others may be new; some may be welcomed, others more critically received; some will require minor adjustments, others will constitute major leaps; some will be stated in full, others will need further development. However, we hope that the ideas and suggestions put forward here will inspire childcare workers, managers and trainers to re-evaluate their theory and practice with the aim to prevent the abuse of women in childcare work in the future.

The way ahead in childcare theory

In this chapter we will rethink childcare theory. We will introduce a new theoretical approach that recognizes the equality of men and women in disciplined, scientific analysis rather than in gender-dominated dogma, opinion or obsession. We have discussed some of the most prevalent traditional childcare theories in Chapter 4. We found that they have a number of things in common. They all try to help workers to identify and describe problems. They aim to help workers to make sense of what is going on. They seek to understand the reasons why people behave the way they do. They intend to help in the prediction of how a client may behave in the future and in the assessment of risk. They usually provide some kind of framework for intervention. But, they have failed to prevent the abuse of women in childcare work. They have failed to protect the mothers of the children that are the focus of childcare workers.

The questions arise: Why have they failed? Why have they not been able to prevent the abuse of women clients? Why have they not provided protection from abuse? Potentially there are a number of reasons why traditional childcare theories have not been able to provide a framework that ensures that clients, in particular women clients, are not abused in childcare work. They have not been used properly. They have not been integrated into practice properly. Or, they have been misunderstood or misapplied. While some of these reasons are responsible for some of the abuse of women in childcare work, most childcare workers probably try to use theories in their work properly and try not to misunderstand or misinterpret theories. It is therefore more likely that something else has caused such a persistent failure to protect women. It is more likely that most of these theories have, in fact, not fully incorporated the abuse of women as an important aspect of their analysis. It is more likely that they have not focused fully on this problem; that they were not sensitive towards issues of gender discrimination; or that they were misleading in their analysis of women's behaviour and/or child development. One thing is sure – these theories have not been able to prevent the abuse described in this book. A re-evaluation is necessary. A non-abusive, gender sensitive theory needs to be developed.

Common sense versus science

It would be nice to be able to introduce a new theoretical approach to childcare work in a few simple words: 'Just use your common sense' 'Just follow your heart', or 'Just go with your gut feeling'. Some people would perhaps welcome such advice. It would confirm their present approach to childcare work which may be based on common beliefs and folk wisdom (see Chapter 5). They would be relieved of the responsibility to look further, to look for a deeper, more complete analysis. However, the majority of childcare workers would not be happy if such advice would be the only thing they can base their practice on. Such advice would also most certainly not protect women clients from abuse. Childcare work is already often criticized as 'lacking clarity of purpose, possessing vagueness of method and showing a wishy-washiness that is altogether indefensible' (Howe 1987: 82). The advice offered above would do nothing to change this. Most childcare workers would probably argue that their practice is not based on common beliefs and proverbs. They may even resent the fact that a book aimed at a professional readership addresses these issues. Common sense and popular beliefs may at times be helpful in solving daily problems. Childcare workers, however, are usually called upon when people are unable to solve their daily problems without professional help. Childcare workers need a more concrete, professional basis.

Childcare workers need a firm base for their practice. They need to know and understand what is going on. They need to be able to identify a problem, to understand and describe it in concrete terms. They need a good theoretical base for assessment and intervention. They need theories that have been well researched and that are based on scientific study. They need these theories to provide them with answers to some of their most fundamental questions: Why do people behave the way they do? For example, why do parents abuse their children? Why do people neglect children? What causes this kind of behaviour? What causes behaviour in general? How can we change behaviour? What can we do to change the behaviour of a parent who is abusive or neglectful? How can we change the behaviour of a child that is out of control, or in danger of hurting themselves or others? How can we predict whether or not someone will pose a risk to a child in future? How can we be sure that the child will be safe at home tonight?

The search for answers

Childcare theories have come a long way in their search for answers. They are widely used to guide childcare practice. However, so far, theories have not provided answers on how best to protect women in childcare work. They have not found answers to how best to prevent such abuse. This problem is not insurmountable. It is a problem which is largely due to the fact that childcare theories have stopped short in their analysis. Theoretical analysis of human conduct, behaviour or development has provided incomplete answers to the key questions: What causes behaviour? How can behaviour be explained? How can behaviour be changed, controlled or predicted? In order to find the step that traditional childcare theories have missed, let us look at the development of childcare theory one step at a time.

Most childcare theories today start by observing human behaviour. Much time and effort is put into observations, or elaborate experimentation is carried out. This research has yielded many results. Much is now known about the sequences of human development. For example, we know which behaviours we can expect to see first in a child and which follow later. Much is known about what people do, when, where and how they do it. How people conduct their lives, how they grow older, how they work, rest and play. This list could obviously be endless. One only has to look into an appropriate textbook to find a wealth of information about human conduct and behaviour. So why have these theories fallen short in the final analysis? Why have they not been able to provide childcare workers with a theory that is sensitive enough to detect and prevent the abuse of women?

The incomplete answer

The main reason why these theories have fallen short in the final analysis is that it is a very difficult job. When theorists were looking for causes of the behaviour that they had observed, they could not find them easily. The complexities of the behaviour were overwhelming. They observed a child throwing a temper tantrum, they observed a parent neglecting a child, they heard a man shouting at his wife, they saw Patricia Murray (Chapter 1) stare at the childcare workers. The crucial questions were: Why do people behave the way they do? Why did the mother neglect her baby? Why did the father abuse his child? Why did the child refuse to go to school? Childcare workers need to know the answers in order to find ways of dealing with these problems.

The search for causes of behaviour began in the place that seemed the obvious first choice: the people themselves. Theorists turned their attention to the people's feelings and thoughts. People felt sad or happy, they felt hurt or frustrated, they felt anxious or relaxed. They thought angry or loving thoughts, they thought of the future or of the past, they thought of other people or of themselves. Oftentimes the thoughts or feelings happened before the person's behaviour could be observed by the researchers. The woman would think angrily about the child and then hit him. The man would feel lovingly towards his wife and then kiss her. The childcare worker would feel scared of the man and then avoid him. The child would think worried thoughts and then play truant. It seemed obvious to conclude that if the thoughts or feelings happened before the behaviour, they must be the cause of the behaviour. Theorists concluded that thoughts or feelings determine what the mother does next, where the father goes, who the childcare worker contacts, when the child returns home.

The short falls

This is usually where the analysis stopped. To all intents and purposes an answer was found. The man hit the woman, because he felt frustrated; the child played truant, because she was scared; the mother stared at the childcare workers because she was angry; the childcare worker avoided the man because she was afraid. Most childcare theories have taken this course. The analysis seemed satisfactory. It seemed as if an answer was found. Thinking and feeling seemed to provide a good enough cause for people to behave the way they do. Some theorists have argued that analysis has to stop somewhere, so this seemed as good a place as any (Killeen (1984) in Hayes and Brownstein 1986). However, leaving the analysis at this point, theories have not prevented the abuse of women in childcare work. The reason for this is two-fold. First, in most cases childcare workers did not actually ask the woman client herself what she was feeling or thinking. They took an educated guess as to what a client was feeling and thinking before she behaved in a certain way. They hypothesized about the feeling or thought that went before the more obvious behaviour. They then relied on their hypothesis when they were looking for a cause of the client's behaviour. When they saw Patricia stare at the childcare workers, they hypothesized that she must be feeling angry, they then concluded that her anger caused her to stare. When they heard the man shout, they hypothesized that he must be feeling frustrated, they concluded that his frustration caused his shouting. When they saw the child missing in school, they hypothesized that he must be feeling scared, they then concluded that his fear caused his truancy. All too often they did not check if their guess was right or wrong.

The presumption, based on traditional childcare theories, was that certain behaviour is caused by certain thoughts or feelings. This presumption is sometimes called 'mentalistic thinking' or 'mentalism' (Hayes and Brownstein 1986; Baum 1994). Childcare workers who rely on a mentalistic analysis try to work out what clients are feeling or thinking in order to establish the cause for client's actions. If in doubt childcare workers hypothesize – that is, guess – and if childcare workers get it wrong, women are misunderstood, misinterpreted, misrepresented, abused.

The more complete answer

Childcare theories in the past have not been able to protect women from the kinds of abuse described in this book because they fell short of a full, detailed, deep analysis. They stopped their analysis when it seemed complete. They stopped because it seems as if they have found an answer, not because they have rigorously pursued all other avenues and came to a standstill. They stopped, not because further analysis would be pointless or impossible. They stopped, not because further experimentation would not yield more detailed results. They simply stopped because they thought they had an answer. This is where their analysis fell short. There are many more questions that need to be answered before a full analysis can be achieved (Malott and Whaley 1983; Poling *et al.* 1990). For example, what caused Patricia to feel the way she did? What caused the man to feel angry? What caused the child to feel scared? What caused Patricia to think angry thoughts? What caused the mother to think loving thoughts? What caused the child to think about avoiding school? If childcare workers really want to understand what causes human behaviour, they need answers to these questions too. If childcare workers want to prevent the abuse of women, they need answers to these questions. They need a full analysis. Hypothetical guessing is no longer good enough. It is far too akin to the common sense advice offered earlier.

Human behaviour redefined

If childcare workers need explanations for the causes of behaviour as well as the causes of feelings and thoughts it makes sense to have another look at thoughts and feelings. What are feelings and thoughts? At the most basic level they are things people do. People 'do' think, they 'do' feel. Consequently, it may be useful to analyse feelings and thoughts by considering them together with other things people do. The usual term for things people do is human behaviour (Skinner 1953). If feelings and thoughts are things people do perhaps we should redefine them as human behaviours (Skinner 1989). With this new definition human behaviour is considered to be 'anything that people do, including what they say and what they think and feel' (Reese *et al.* 1978: 2). With this definition of behaviour childcare workers can now look at the causes of human behaviour in a much more holistic sense. When internal feelings and thoughts are considered human behaviour, childcare workers no longer rely on hypothetical guesses about feelings and thoughts when they are looking for causes of behaviour. They are now looking at the man's hitting and the angry feelings that accompany the hitting and wonder what caused both of these behaviours. They realize that one behaviour may follow another, but that one behaviour cannot be the cause of another behaviour. The angry feelings may come first and then the hitting. However, the cause of 'feeling' behaviour cannot be found in 'hitting' behaviour. With this redefinition childcare workers realize that causes have to be found for both kinds of behaviour. They have to re-evaluate old ways of analysis and rethink old theories.

Science of behaviour

Scientists have, of course, struggled with the kind of issues discussed here for a long time. Finding the cause of human behaviour has been the arena of psychology for centuries. Many psychologists have been searching for causes of behaviour inside the person by hypothesizing about their thought and feelings. We have discussed the shortcomings of this approach. One branch of psychology, however, has gone the other way. In this branch of psychology scientists were also looking for the causes of behaviour. However, they were not looking inside the person, they were looking 'outside'. This branch is based on the science of behaviour called behaviour analysis (Skinner 1989).

The science of behaviour is not entirely new to childcare workers (Pinkston *et al.* 1982; Herbert 1986; Howe 1987; Hudson and McDonald 1991). For example, it is used in change and modifying problem behaviours in specialized, residential, and field work settings. The client group which benefits most from the application of the knowledge gained through a scientific analysis of behaviour are usually those with learning difficulties or those with extreme or otherwise unchangeable behaviour problems. When applied properly and thoroughly the effects can be astounding. Self-injurious behaviour can be halted; clients who were diagnosed as autistic can be taught to behave pro-socially; anorexic girls can be seen eating again; chronic enuresis can be cured (Martin and Pear 1992). Examples of successful application of behaviour analysis can be found in many professional or academic journals and books (for example, *Journal of Applied Behaviour Analysis*; *Research in Social Work Practice*; Gragiano 1971; Mash *et al.* 1976; Herbert 1978, 1989; Beck and Barlow 1984; Gelfand and Hartman 1986). The question arises, if this approach is so successful in the most difficult situations, could it be used to benefit women who are abused in childcare work? Can it offer a non-abusive, gender-sensitive theoretical approach to childcare work as a whole? Can it help childcare workers who want to protect women and children from the kind of abuse described in this book? Let's find out.

The analysis of behaviour

The first benefit of a behaviour analytic approach to the abuse of women in childcare work is that the feelings, thoughts and actions that characterize this abuse are considered and analysed as human behaviour. The term abuse of women is viewed as a descriptive term for a complex combination of behaviours. We have seen many examples of the complexities of abuse of women in childcare work throughout this book. However, on the most basic level the abuse of women in childcare work is the behaviour of those involved in the system, clients as well as workers. We have discussed earlier (Chapter 3) that people have to learn how to behave in relationships. Clients learn how to relate to workers and workers learn how to relate to clients. A complex network of relationships develops when relationships apart from the client–worker relationships are considered. The behaviour of each person in this complex network is affected by the behaviour of the others.

When childcare workers consider the relationships they have with clients in terms of behaviour, the abuse of women can be redefined in this way too. It can then be analysed by using the findings of behaviour analysis. As mentioned earlier, this analysis has concentrated on finding the causes of behaviour 'outside' the behaviour in question. Behaviour analysts do not look for the cause of Patricia's stare in her fear or anger. They view her feelings as part of her behaviour. They look for the cause of her stare and her fearful or angry feelings outside of Patricia's behaviour – for example, the appearance of the childcare workers and Patricia's previous experience with them. This kind of analysis offers a different, deeper and more constructive analysis to childcare theory, because now childcare workers are able to do something about the situation. When they were still looking for the cause of Patricia's stare in her feelings and made educated guesses as to what these may be, their hands were tied. They had reached the end of their analysis. Now, they realize that her feelings as well as her actions were caused by outside factors, such as, for example, the appearance of childcare workers. They can now proactively work at changing these factors and at achieving non-abusive practices.

Behaviour analysis and childcare work

The second advantage of a behaviour analytic approach to childcare work is that it offers an approach which is firmly based in sound scientific principles: 'This is the first time that [an analysis of] human problems has been based on experimentally obtained information rather than on personal speculation or opinion' (Deibert and Harmon 1978: 6). The scientific approach to behaviour started with careful experimentation in the laboratories of experimental psychologists. The first findings were made nearly accidentally, but soon scientific rigour characterized the field (for example, once Pavlov had accidentally discovered the basic principle of classical conditioning he then used rigorous experiments to identify what exactly was going on). Careful experimentation led to the discovery of some very basic principles (such as habituation, classical conditioning, operant conditioning, extinction, shaping, etc.). These principles are basic facts, and yet so universal, that they are often considered laws of behaviour: 'In fact, some of these principles are so basic that they have taken on the status of a law' (Deibert and Harmon 1978: 6).

Most childcare workers are familiar with these principles or behavioural laws, but as mentioned earlier, they usually refer to them only when treating extreme problem behaviours. They do not always realize that these principles are in operation even when they are not consciously aware of it. Laws of behaviour, like laws of physics or biology, are operating even if they are not fully understood. Take for example, the heart. A person does not have to understand all the medical or biological facts for their heart to beat and keep them alive. Of course, if the heart causes a problem because it is not working properly, only a person who understands the medical or biological facts can help. The basic laws or principles of behaviour operate similarly. They are working whether we understand them or not. However, if behaviour causes problems, a person who understands behavioural laws and principles can help. In the context discussed here the problem behaviour is when women are abused in childcare work. A full understanding of the laws responsible for the behaviour enables childcare workers to help and prevent abuse or protect women clients and their children: 'Ignorance of these facts is a luxury we can no longer afford' (Reese *et al.* 1978: 8).

Basic principles of behaviour

The third benefit of a behavioural analysis in childcare work is that, as mentioned earlier, the analysis concentrates on factors outside of the behaviour itself. The analysis concentrates mainly on the context in which the behaviour occurs and the consequences which follow the behaviour. The technical term for this relationship is 'contingency'. We will try and avoid technical terms in this chapter mainly because most childcare workers are not really interested in technical jargon. They are usually too preoccupied with practical matters. However, any science has its own vocabulary. For example, most of us would probably not understand a word if we heard two astrophysicists talking to each other. The two astrophysicists, however, would not be able to talk about the specifics of their science if they could not use clearly and precisely defined terms. This does not mean that they are not concerned with practical matters. They too want to solve practical problems. It is therefore sometimes necessary to clearly define terms in science.

The term 'contingency' is at the centre of behaviour analysis, in particular the term A-B-C-contingency. This term refers to the causal relationship between the context in which a behaviour occurs (the **A**ntecedent), the **B**ehaviour itself, and the **C**onsequences that follow the behaviour. In this relationship the behaviour is the dependent variable. Behaviour change depends on changes of either the context or the consequences. In brief, behaviour changes and adapts to the contingencies that are in operation at any given time (Holland 1978). Let us look at examples. Childcare workers are familiar with behaviour changes. They observe a child at home and later they observe the same child in the office. The behaviour of the child is usually different. The behaviour of the child changed when the context changed. Or, childcare workers observe a child tidying up and consequently being praised, later, maybe the next day, they observe the same child tidying up again. The consequences influenced the behaviour of the child. The easiest way to stop the child from tidying up in the future is to reprimand him for tidying up today. Changing context or consequences means changing behaviour. As Holland (1978) put it, 'It takes changed contingencies to change behavior' (p. 34).

Contingency analysis

The aim of this chapter is to find a theory that enables childcare workers to change the behaviours that lead to the abuse of women. Childcare workers need to find the best and most effective way to change this behaviour. We have seen that behaviour is determined by the context in which it occurs and by the consequences which follow. We have called the relationship between **A**ntecedent context, **B**ehaviour and **C**onsequence 'contingency'. Behaviour analytic research has shown that it takes changed contingencies to change behaviour. It follows that, if abuse of women is behaviour, and it takes changed contingencies to change behaviour, the best way to change the abuse of women is to change the contingencies that are responsible for it. If we want to prevent the abuse of women in childcare work we have to change either the context in which the abuse happens or the consequences which follow the abuse. Many questions arise. What are the consequences? What is the context of abuse? And, how can we change them? In this section we will look at each of these questions.

Obviously the contingencies which are responsible for the abuse of women in childcare work are complex and complicated. The best way to analyse them is to take them one at a time and look at how each aspect functions on the behaviour in question. This kind of analysis is called 'functional analysis'. Functional analysis is a relatively recent development in childcare work (National Institute for Social Work 1994) and is used for the precise measurement of the contingencies responsible for the development and maintenance of behaviour (Neef 1994). Functional analysis has many benefits. Properly carried out, functional analysis offers a full, holistic picture of the client's situation. It helps the worker to identify the contingencies responsible for certain behaviours. It reminds the worker that the client's behaviour is a result of his/her experiences. It ensures that the worker assesses past experiences as well as present context. And, it leads the way towards effective intervention (Van Houten *et al.* 1988; Johnston and Sherman 1993).

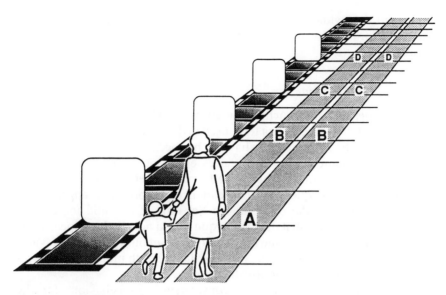

Figure 10.1 Behavioural stream
Reprinted with permission. M. Keenan (1991)

In functional analysis workers remember that their meeting with clients happens within the context of clients' lives and that the workers' behaviour functions as a consequence for the clients' behaviour and vice versa. This continuous behavioural interchange has been called the 'behavioural stream' (Keenan 1991, 1993). The term is used to illustrate that behaviour never stops and is continuously influenced by its context and consequences. The worker meets the client during a 'snapshot' in the continuum of the client's life experiences. Figure 10.1 illustrates how the idea of the behavioural stream can be conceptualized. The figure shows a mother and her child walking along the continuum of their life experiences. The letters on their path represent different experiences. The frames on the film strip represent snapshots in time. The childcare worker meets with mother and child at any one of these frames. Childcare referral, assessment, investigation, or intervention takes place. The meeting constitutes an experience for the mother and child, it has consequences for mother and child (and childcare workers, of course). After the meeting the mother, child and childcare worker move on to the next experience.

Using Figure 10.1 as conceptual guide, we will now look at each of the components that constitute a functional analysis. Dealing with each component separately may appear fragmented. However, it is important to analyse each step on the way to enable workers to find out exactly where the problem lies, which aspect of their behaviour constitutes an abusive experience for the mother, what constitutes an abusive context. It is important that while workers do this they do not lose sight of the whole picture. Workers always have to remember the complexity of the whole process.

Consequences of behaviour

The first question in a functional analysis is: What are consequences of behaviour? 'Consequence' is a term used to describe a vast range of things. Anything that happens *after* a behaviour has occurred can be considered a consequence. Sometimes consequences even appear long after the behaviour is finished. They still have an effect on the behaviour. For example, the monthly pay cheque is the consequence of working. It appears long after the first working day of the month. Yet, most of us would not work on the first day of the month if the pay cheque would not reliably appear at the end. In a sense the pay cheque is a consequence of our working behaviour on the first (and all subsequent) working days of each month and ensures that we continue to work month after month.

What is the use of discussing consequences of behaviour for the prevention of abuse of women? The reason why it is important to be aware of the consequences of behaviour is that they have different effects on the behaviour. Some consequences make behaviour more frequent, stronger, more vigorous, or longer lasting; others make behaviour less frequent, weaker, less vigorous, or they make behaviour disappear altogether. If childcare workers want to change client behaviours – for example, behaviours such as feeling abused, thinking resentful or fearful thoughts, saying insulting things, or acting aggressively, and make them appear less frequently, less vigorously or disappear altogether – they need to understand the consequences that have led to the client behaviour in the first place. By changing the consequences, the behaviour will change. If childcare workers want to encourage client behaviours such as participation, cooperation, feeling supported, thinking caring thoughts, and acting responsibly they need to understand the consequences which will lead to an increase of this behaviour.

What are these consequences? At this point we need two more technical terms because there are two different kinds of consequences. Technically and scientifically they are termed according to their effect on the behaviour. The consequences which lead to 'more' behaviours are called 'reinforcers'. Consequences which lead to 'less' behaviour are called 'punishers'. Both of these terms are defined by their function, the effect they have on the behaviour. This all sounds very technical. Let us look at it in practice. Patricia Murray in Chapter 1 was clearly abused by the childcare workers who visited her. During the early part of the childcare workers' visit, we observed that Patricia frequently protested and asserted herself, at one point she even 'erupted' and yelled at the childcare workers.

Later Patricia became rather quiet. She could 'barely respond'. She just 'wished that she could be alone'. We observed a drastic change of Patricia's behaviour. Why did Patricia's behaviour change so drastically? The behaviour analytic answer lies in an analysis of the consequences of Patricia's assertive behaviour. The consequence for Patricia's assertive behaviour, was the behaviour of the childcare workers. Their comments, looks, questions and interrogations had an effect on Patricia's behaviour. It changed. She became quiet and non-assertive, she felt intimidated, scared, frightened, helpless and abused. Her assertive behaviours were effectively 'punished'.

What would have been the alternative? Could her behaviour have been 'reinforced'? Clearly the response of the childcare workers had an effect on Patricia's behaviour. If childcare workers are fully aware of the effect of their own behaviour on client behaviour they realize that they can control this effect. Childcare workers can (and do) reinforce client behaviour. It does not depend on whether they are aware of it or not. In Patricia's case they unwittingly and unintentionally reinforced behaviour (remember this includes feelings and thoughts) that can be described as frightened, intimidated and abused. They could have reinforced behaviours that are more helpful and less abusing. They could have reinforced protective, supportive, caring, loving, cooperative and assertive behaviours. If they had concentrated on reinforcing these kind of behaviours their job would probably have been much easier and Patricia would not have felt abused. Let us recap briefly. Consequences follow behaviour and have an effect on behaviour. They either increase or decrease behaviour. They have this effect whether we know about it or not. Childcare workers who understand the effects of consequences on behaviour should use this knowledge to reinforce appropriate behaviours in clients. Clients treated this way do not experience abuse.

Context of behaviour

We have discussed the importance of consequences in a functional analysis of the abuse of women in childcare work. While consequences play an important part, there are obviously other factors that are important. A full analysis includes looking at consequences and the context of the behaviour in question. The next question is therefore: What is the context of abuse? 'Context' is a term used for the situation in which a behaviour occurs, the stimuli to which a person responds, or the cue that lies in the situation. People behave differently in different situations. Parents are often surprised when they see their child in a new situation, for example, in a neighbour's house or in school. Children behave differently in different situations. They behave assertively in one situation, quietly in another. The same is obviously true for adults. They behave differently in different situations: in buses, they sit; in queues, they stand; in conversations, they talk; in churches, they are silent. The question is what determines how people behave in each of these situations.

The answer to this question brings us back to the effect of consequences on behaviour, because people learn to behave differently in different situations depending on the consequences they have experienced in these situations. Behaviour that may be punished (decreased) in one situation, may be reinforced (increased) in another. This way the context becomes an important cue and people behave accordingly. We have seen earlier that behaviour is adaptable. Behaviour adapts to different situations. This phenomenon has been called 'stimulus control'. The importance of understanding stimulus control in childcare work becomes apparent when we take, for example, Patricia Murray's response to the social workers at her door. She 'suddenly' felt uneasy, anxious and resentful. Given our analysis so far, this response should not surprise. Patricia's behaviour may well have been shaped by her previous experiences with the childcare workers. Certain behaviours may have been reinforced, others punished and therefore seeing childcare workers presented the context which controlled Patricia's behaviour. Understanding stimulus control helps childcare workers predict client responses. Childcare workers can therefore predict feelings of abuse or intimidation in advance and should ensure that the context provides non-abusive cues for clients.

Imitation and modelling

The analysis of consequences and context is important in a re-evaluation of childcare theory. But what about the behaviour of others? For example, we have explained Patricia's behaviour by looking at the behaviour of childcare workers. In this case the behaviour of the childcare workers provided context and consequences to Patricia's behaviour. Clearly human behaviour does not happen in isolation. People relate to one another all the time. The abuse of women in childcare work does not happen in isolation, it happens in a social context. People learn much of their behaviour either by watching others or by listening to them. In this section of this chapter we will look at the effects of other people's behaviour on the abused client, Patricia, and suggest ways how this new understanding can be used to prevent abuse.

Patricia's response to childcare workers was predictable, if she had met the workers before. But, what if this was the first time Patricia had met the childcare workers? What if they had not been instrumental in shaping her behaviour? In this case it is possible that another principle of behaviour was at work: imitation learning or 'modelling'. Patricia may have seen neighbours responding to childcare workers who called at their door or she may have seen television programmes in which childcare workers took children into care. Patricia may have modelled her behaviour on others. People learn much of their behaviour from others and the fact that they can learn by imitating others is probably responsible for much of civilization.

However, imitation learning is not just straightforward. The ability to imitate has to be learnt first (Baer *et al.* 1967). The ability to imitate is usually learnt very young. Some babies seem to imitate nearly from birth and many games parents play with their baby are aimed at improving the baby's ability to imitate. If the ability to imitate is shaped and reinforced successfully, people can learn rapidly from each other. Childcare workers can (and do) use client's ability to imitate in their work quite successfully. The success of imitation learning usually depends on the observer's ability to imitate. It also depends on the model. The model's similarity to the observer, the model's competence, the observer's previous experience with the model, the model's prestige and the use of multiple models all increase the success of imitation learning (Sulzer-Azaroff and Mayer 1991).

Childcare workers can use modelling to teach clients childcare skills, parenting skills, home management, skills, etc. They can also use modelling in preparing parents for parental participation in childcare conferences or other decision making forums. Childcare workers must take into consideration that clients will at times model on them even if this is not planned. For example, when childcare workers do not turn up for meetings or continuously cancel appointments at the last moment, clients may imitate this behaviour and, for example, cancel appointments with health visitors or doctors or not attend childcare conferences. All too often clients are then considered irresponsible or unreliable and childcare workers get 'concerned about the mother's commitment to her child's health and well-being' without reference to the possible effect of modelling. Childcare workers are usually not held responsible for their irresponsible and unreliable behaviour when cancelling client appointments. Childcare workers who use modelling carefully can teach loving, caring, assertive and cooperative skills, and will be experienced by clients as supportive, caring and non-abusive.

Say-do correspondence and interviewing clients

Imitation learning is one way in which people learn from each other, language is another. People learn vast amounts by listening to what others say or reading what others have written. For example, Patricia may have heard her neighbours talk about their experiences with childcare workers or she may have read about the misconduct of childcare workers in child abuse cases in the newspapers. Her response to the childcare workers at her door may have been influenced by what she had heard or read. Childcare workers usually rely on the spoken word in their assessment as well as in their intervention.

However, the effect of the spoken or the written word is not as predictable or reliable as is often expected. An increasing number of research studies found that people do not reliably do what they say they do (Lloyd 1994a, 1994b). This is not unfamiliar to childcare workers or clients. Much is said, promised, agreed, verbally contracted or negotiated in childcare work. This does not always mean that corresponding actions will follow. This lack of correspondence between what is said and what is done can be frustrating for both clients and workers.

It seems obvious that what people say and how they say it depends on the context in which they speak and the consequences of what is said. For example, when the childcare workers asked Patricia, 'How might Carl react?', they wanted to assess the risk for the children. However, they were relying on Patricia's verbal prediction of Carl's reaction. Patricia's response to the question must be viewed in the context in which this question was asked. We have seen earlier that this context caused anxious and angry thoughts and feelings for Patricia. It is likely that her verbal response would also reflect the context. Her response must also be viewed in the light of the likely consequences of her answer. If she says the wrong thing her children may be taken into care. By asking this question the childcare workers put Patricia into an impossible situation. Even if she is worried about Carl's reaction, she cannot express her worry in fear of the consequences. The childcare workers were going to rely on Patricia's statement about Carl's reaction in their decision making and in their assessment of whether or not the children were safe at home. Their assessment of Patricia's ability to cope would also be based on her response. Childcare workers must analyse the context and the consequences of a client's verbal behaviour before asking unrealistic questions. Their reliance on the answers can only be experienced as abusive by clients

Further exploration of non-abusive childcare theory

In the previous paragraphs we have looked at some of the basic principles of behaviour analysis. We used this approach to analyse the abuse of women in childcare work and establish how this approach can be used to prevent this kind of abuse in future. What is offered here is obviously only a tentative and rather brief treatise of this theoretical approach. Human behaviour is extremely complex and a full analysis would require much more space than is available here. Interested readers are therefore invited to consult the following authors for detailed analysis of a wide range of topics which are relevant to childcare workers. For example, Wheeler

(1973) and Sidman (1989) used behaviour analysis to analyse the effects of coercive systems in detail; other kinds of social behaviour were thoroughly analysed from a behavioural perspective by Guerin (1994); Lundin (1969) provided a behaviour analysis of the term 'personality'; behaviour analysis of language and cognition was recently offered by Hayes *et al.* (1994); thinking and feeling and self-control were behaviourally analysed by Reese *et al.* (1978); loss and bereavement were behaviourally analysed by Dillenburger and Keenan (1994b); women's sexuality, domestic violence and rape, and sex roles were analysed and methods of effective intervention suggested in a book edited by Beck and Barlow (1984). Child development and childcare issues figure prominently in behaviour analysis literature. For example, a behaviour analysis of child development was offered by Baer and his colleagues (Baer 1970, 1973; Rosales and Baer in press), Bijou (1993) and Morris *et al.* (1982); attachment behaviours were analysed by Gewirtz and his colleagues (Gewirtz and Boyd 1977; Gewirtz 1991; Gewirtz and Kurtines 1991; Gewirtz and Peláez-Nogueras 1991, 1992); child rearing practices based on behavioural principles were suggested by Dillenburger and Keenan (1994a); and developmental disabilities and ethical codes of practice were addressed within a behavioural framework by Hayes *et al.* (1994). Guidance to a vast variety of applications of behaviour analysis is provided by Cooper *et al.* (1987) and Sulzer-Azaroff and Mayer (1991).

For readers who are completely new to the behavioural approach and who are not familiar with the basic principles of behaviour, Millenson and Leslie (1979) give a detailed overview of the history and basic experimental findings, and Baldwin and Baldwin (1986), Rachlin (1991), Catania (1992), Malott *et al.* (1993) and Grant and Evans (1994) describe the basic, elementary principles of behaviour. Basic introductory texts were provided by Deibert and Harmon (1978) and Pryor (1984).

Conclusion

In this chapter a theoretical approach to childcare work has been introduced that aims to prevent the abuse of women in childcare work. Traditional theories were evaluated and it was found that they often base their explanations on hypothetical presumptions and guesswork about internal causes. This does not offer a firm, scientific basis for childcare work and does not prevent the abusive practices. A thorough rethink of childcare theory was necessary. In this chapter behaviour analysis was introduced as a sensitive, thoroughly researched and precisely defined approach that can usefully be applied in childcare work. Behaviour analysis begins by defining behaviour. A behaviour analytical definition of behaviour differs from traditional definitions in that thinking, feeling, speaking and acting are all considered behaviours in need of explanation. The causes for these behaviours are sought in the prevailing contingencies.

We have discussed the benefits of a full functional analysis of the contingencies that are responsible for the abuse of women in childcare work. We have offered examples of such an analysis for some of the issues that were abusive in Patricia Murray's case (Chapter 1). Figure 10.1 was included to offer a graphic representation of the conceptual issues involved in a functional analysis. The functional behaviour analytic approach offers a new, thorough, non-abusive approach to childcare work. Moreover, it offers an effective set of interventions which have successfully been applied in a vast variety of problem situations and which have been thoroughly and scientifically researched.

11

Non-abusive childcare systems

Introduction

This chapter will focus upon the various components of abusive childcare systems, and suggest alternative ways in which the abuse can be minimized. The term 'minimizing abuse' may provoke some readers, who believe that childcare workers and the systems in which they work should eradicate all forms of abuse of clients, irrespective of its degree or its extent. But the authors have from the outset attempted some confrontation themselves; confronting reality that is, the reality of certain characteristics of childcare systems and individuals that are so entrenched and/or pervasive, and which are initiated and/or supported and sustained by so many vested interests, that they are not easily going to be transformed in the way necessary for the total abolition of abuse against women. For example, we realize that childcare workers themselves can do very little about what is probably the most woman-abusive feature of childcare agencies (particularly social services), namely, the constant and pervasive changes being imposed on those agencies (see Chapter 6 for the precise details of how this constant change can lead to the abuse of mothers in particular).

Despite the lesson learnt, primarily through enquiry reports, that massive changes in the structure and organization of childcare agencies pose major risks to childcare services and to the welfare of the primary carers of children, both government and management seem determined to inflict more and more massive changes upon those agencies. Substantial progress can be made, however, in many of the other components of abusive childcare systems. First, such systems can become immune and resistant to abusive, prevailing, political climates, and to the abusive legislation which may stem from the same. Second, exposing the abusive potential of existing legislation, in particular the Children Act. Some sections have been blatantly misinterpreted and exploited, and many women abused as a consequence. Amendments are inevitable, and managers and frontline staff can make a valuable contribution to the debate preceding those amendments. Third, staff can be supervised and monitored more effectively to ensure that women clients are not the victims of staff's obsessive convictions, nor of staff's own past experiences of victimization. Fourth, managers of childcare agencies can free themselves and their workforces from the blanket no-risk policies and procedures which concentrate and wreak so much havoc upon single mothers in particular, and, ultimately, upon children themselves. Fifth, policies and procedures can be modified or replaced to give mothers a much better deal in such areas as: referral and investigation (ensuring that non-abusing mothers are not treated as though they were perpetrators); domestic violence (confronting the woman's predicament rather than ignoring it); ensuring men are not avoided and women exploited as a consequence of that avoidance; and parental participation. This chapter will look at each of these components and suggest a way forward; as always, the authors will retain a firm grip on the realities of practice, and of the complexities and difficulties in the tasks of both practitioners and managers.

Resisting the abusive political climate

Western societies and their political institutions remain as capable as they always have been of developing negative, destructive perceptions of particular groups of people, and enacting laws which, in application, will be abusive to those people. Numerous examples of the process were provided in Chapter 6, and it is coincidental that these words are being written precisely on the day that the British Prime Minister John Major has caused a national furore by his attack on beggars (*Bristol Evening News*, 27 May 1994). Whether he intended to or not, he has generated an abusive climate against a totally powerless group of people. Meanwhile, his ministers, notably Peter Lilley, Secretary of State for Social Security, continue with their campaign against single parent mothers. His speech of 20 June 1994, alarmed even the *Daily Mail*, the editor of which felt obliged to devote two whole pages to single parent mothers who wanted to protest about the speech (*Daily Mail*, 22 June 1994). Frontline professionals may be depressed at the realization that they have no control over these potentially destructive utterances by politicians, nor the scapegoating of single parent mothers which may result (or any group which politicians feel is ripe for picking on to gain some popularity and votes). Much more serious, however, is when politicians' prejudices or opportunism progresses to discriminatory legislation and/or procedures and guidelines.

O'Hagan (1989) recalled the impact on frontline workers of many of the damaging guidelines and procedures implemented by all the relevant agencies during the anti-child sexual abuse crusade of 1986–8 (upon which prominent politicians were riding). The first obligation, therefore, is to scrutinize new procedures and guidelines and to identify any potential for abuse. This is not merely the duty of managers; it is everyone's duty, as ethically sound as it is professionally enriching. We may consider it in relation to (1) certain sections of the 1989 Children Act; (2) the policy of 'ousting' men believed to constitute a threat to children; (3) the Child Support Agency; and (4) the Government's repeal of the Homeless Person's Act.

The Children Act

In Chapter 6, reference was made to the potentially abusive features of the Children Act. These included tighter control and surveillance of single parent mothers; a lack of financial provision enabling local authorities to adhere to its principles on prevention; its effect of increasing the adversarial nature of care proceedings; its advocacy of partnership with parents, yet not spelling this out (consequently 'partnership' being implemented in whatever way local authorities see fit), etc. One may look in more detail at the Act and find specific sections which make abuse almost inevitable. Take section 34, for example, on parental contact: 'Where a child is in the care of the local authority, the authority shall (subject to the provisions of this section) allow the child reasonable contact with (a) his parents...'. Preceding the Act, the prevention of contact was a common abuse perpetrated against mothers. These opening words in section 34, are therefore welcome. However, in subsection 6(a), the Act states that the local authority may refuse contact, if they are 'satisfied that it is necessary to do so in order to safeguard or promote the child's welfare'. The Act does not specify the grounds necessary for feeling satisfied, and there is a real danger of some individual managers and practitioners drifting towards an exploitation of the enormous discretionary power of this section.

Similarly, with the duty of a local authority to inform parents of the whereabouts of their child – a basic principle one might think, worthy of much effort to uphold. But paragraph 15 of Schedule 2 permits the same potentially abusive discretion when it states: 'Nothing ... requires a local authority to inform any person of the whereabouts of a child if: (a) the child is in the care of the Authority; and: the authority has reasonable cause to believe that informing the person would prejudice the child's welfare'. Again, there is no specification on what constitutes 'reasonable cause', and some parents are obviously cowed into submission by the mere utterance of this particular section (Jackson 1993). Childcare legislation is always open to interpretation and will always contain potentially abusive elements; the recognition of them is an important requisite for the commitment to avoid exploiting the potential.

'Ousting' men without abusing women

When professionals have good reason to suspect that a man is a potential child abuser, it is perfectly laudable to aim to remove that man from any children with whom he resides. Yet, as has been suggested in previous chapters, men and women have been victimized by this aim, the former subjected to persistent harrying, the latter subjected to blatant threats. Our experiences, and the literature to which we have referred (for example, PAIN 1990b; Hooper 1992; Howitt 1992) convinces us that 'ousting' men by threatening women with the removal of their children, is common practice throughout the British Isles. We also believe this unprincipled and ultimately damaging practice is usually carried out by avoiding the man in question; all the efforts and pressures exerted by professionals are directed against the woman. Such was the case detailed by Hayes (1992), of *R* v. *Devon County Council*. At no time did any childcare professional attempt to interview Mr R. They merely descended upon the women who had taken him in and warned of dire consequences, that is, care proceedings in respect of their children. There are professionals who, regrettably, believe there is nothing wrong with this practice; that it is in the best interests of the child; that the right (and duty) to work like this is enshrined in the Children Act, and that the judgment made in the case of Mr R. in favour of the Council, confirms this. Herein lies a guarantee that childcare systems will remain abusive.

The risk of abuse by the man in question may be minimized by getting him removed, but the pressures and threats brought to bear upon the mother inevitably reduce the quality of care she provides for the child. Furthermore, repeatedly avoiding the man and pressurizing the woman to get the man removed creates dangers for that woman. As in the case described by Hayes, such practice was counterproductive: two of the women who took Mr R. in, and who were obviously angry at workers demanding they get him out, managed to dupe the workers into thinking that he had gone; they had in fact managed to conceal his continuing stay for a considerable period. It is a major folly to believe that the Children Act permits threats made against women in promotion of a policy of 'ousting' men; but it is easy to see how the relevant section of the Act has been misinterpreted and corrupted to defend the practice. Paragraph 2 of Schedule 5 states that the suspected abuser who 'proposes to move' may be assisted by the Authority, either financially or otherwise. It says nothing more and nothing less pertinent on the matter. The widespread practice of ousting men by threatening women has, therefore, no legal, professional nor ethical mandate (despite the judgment in *R* v. *Devon County Council*, in which the threats made against mothers was not an issue). The gap between the laudable aim of assisting suspected abusers to move and the reality of what is happening throughout the country to women residing with them is such that urgent action needs to be taken is respect of the above part of the Act. It requires one of those many qualifying or warning paragraphs liberally scattered through its pages, hinged to the main sections; something to the effect that: 'the authority may assist the person suspected, to move from the child's home ... etc., but, **nothing in this section permits the coercion of, or threats directed against, a mother who is residing with the suspected person'.**

The Child Support Act/Agency

Throughout the period in which this book has been written, a major battle has been, and still is being, fought out between (1) powerful pressure groups representing, in the main, male victims of the CSA and supported by many highly influential male politicians and newspaper editors, and (2) single parent mothers supported by much less powerful, less influential pressure groups. It is likely that by the time this book is published the battle will have been won by the former (newspaper editors will hail a victory for common sense and reasonableness), and the legislation which set up the agency will have been so substantially amended, that even the principle that absent fathers should maintain their children, may be compromised. The point was made in Chapter 6 that the real plight of many poor, unsupported, inarticulate, single mothers and their vulnerability to the interrogations of CSA officers, have been lost in this ferocious struggle between the opposing forces of the debate; it may well turn out that it is precisely this particular sector of women who end up as the main victims of whatever solutional amendments are made. In the CSA's first annual report (released 4 July 1994), it revealed that nearly 700 women were recommended for a reduction in benefit as a consequence of the interviews conducted by CSA officers. The most recent and damning confirmation of the CSA's adverse impact upon poor single parent mothers is the research commissioned by 5 national children's organizations (Clarke, Glendinning and Craig, 1994). They concluded that the lone mothers had failed to benefit in any of the ways predicted by the government: '. . . lone mothers reported very high levels of anxiety and stress which had been triggered by the prospect of Agency intervention and by the uncertainties surrounding the progress of their own particular cases. The impact of this anxiety on the children . . . is immeasurable' (p. 113).

Childcare professionals working with any mothers being investigated by the CSA should, if the mothers so wish, be present during the interviews. They should be willing to intervene if the questioning becomes oppressive or sexist. If it does, they should record this and complain through the proper channels. They should represent, or seek someone else to represent, and support mothers through any appeals tribunal.

Such support and advocacy may become more prominent in the future. It is not beyond the bounds of probability that if pressure groups and their influential male political allies succeed in substantially weakening the Agency and its functions (as now seems likely), then CSA officers may feel even less inhibited in their treatment of the poorest, most inarticulate, most unsupported and isolated single mothers. The officers' principal function will remain, irrespective of whatever amendments are made – that is, to save money for the Treasury; to gain evidence and information which will enable them to save money. The prospects for these single mothers are bleak, and childcare agencies, both management and frontline staff, need to prepare.

Repeal of the Homeless Person's Act

Chapter 6 referred to expert opinion on the consequences of repealing the Homeless Person's Act. The Presbyterian Church and no less than seven leading childcare charities launched a campaign to persuade the Government not to repeal (*The Times*, 13 July 1994). They warned of the consequences, particularly for one parent families with very young children. The government went ahead with the repeal and is now attempting to enlighten local authority housing departments and childcare agencies as to the 'merits' of the new legislation. Again, managers and frontline workers in childcare agencies need to scrutinize, identify, expose and record all evidence of hardship attributable to the repeal. There will be, as predicted, plenty of such evidence in respect of single parent mothers and their children. It should not be forgotten that the new legislation was hastily formulated during a virulent anti-single parent mother campaign, orchestrated by leading members of the Government. It is inevitable, therefore, as predicted by so many childcare agencies, that single parent mothers have been targeted.

Childcare workers have a role in contributing to the evidence about the impact of the repeal. They are ideally placed to monitor and record the emotional and psychological repercussions on very young children subjected to continuous moves from one inadequate accommodation to another. They are perfectly within their rights to convey what they see and know to the appropriate housing bodies. Childcare managers and their staff may be right in thinking that, like everyone else, they are helpless to prevent discriminatory legislation that has its origins in the prejudices and emotions of party political conferences. But they are certainly not powerless in exposing such legislation, and may add to the groundswell of public and professional opinion which will bring about necessary change. Cleveland (Butler-Sloss 1988) has some lessons here: groups of significant workers (for example, nurses and emergency duty staff) did realize how abusive services were becoming as a result of new directives, which in turn were the result of a not very intelligent, highly emotional, anti-child sexual abuse crusade; those groups did record and they did protest, and they were eventually heard.

Clarifying motivation

Chapter 5 exposed a number of potentially abusive motivating factors such as: (1) traditional beliefs; (2) personal convictions; (3) gut instincts; and (4) painful past experiences. Professionals motivated by such factors are not always aware of them; indeed they may mistake them for sound ethical principles, applicable and tested theory, good professional practice (Sommerfeld and Hughes 1987; Black *et al.* 1993). Some examples of the first three of the factors included: 'mothers can cope with almost any difficulty, pressure, or strain'; 'men are not worth bothering about'; 'grandmothers know better', etc. Examples of item 4 – that is, painful past experiences – included: being professionally responsible for a child during the time he or she was injured or killed (thereby leading to rigid, risk-free, potentially parent-abusing approaches and practices in all future childcare cases); deprivations, abuses, or destructive relationships in one's own past leading to inappropriate attitudes and/or damaging projections onto significant persons (particularly mothers) in existing cases. It should be stressed that very few, if any, workers are *not* influenced in their work, positively and negatively, by significant events in their past. The problem arises when such events become a negative motivating factor that is clearly harmful to the therapeutic or intervention process, and neither worker nor manager is aware of it. There are two major tasks for management in countering these potentially abusive motivating factors. First, to ensure they they are aware. Awareness should ideally be achieved in professional training (see Chapter 12), but occasionally, as is evident in some of the case histories, workers successfully qualify without them or their trainers ever having addressed the matter. Managers need to keep that possibility in mind in the initial interviewing and vetting of staff, and later in supervision and monitoring. Second, senior managers must ensure that no policy or procedure can be (mis)interpreted as supporting any of these potentially abusive motivating factors.

Non-abusive policy and procedure

The welfare principle

The welfare principle, in all its clarity and simplicity, remains central in childcare policy and procedure. Yet time and time again we have seen this principle transformed into an instrument of abuse itself. Policy makers and managers have to be aware of how and when this is done (see Chapter 5). The most common way is to grossly exaggerate perceived differences or conflict between the welfare of the child and the rights of the parent; there is, far more often, much greater difference and conflict between the welfare of the child and the alternative care provided by underfunded, resourceless childcare agencies. Policy documents and agency procedures should highlight the fact that, despite its simplicity and clarity, the welfare principle is the source of enormous complexity and difficulty to those who have to apply it. More importantly, they should contain comprehensive criteria enabling workers to adhere to the principle, enabling them to plot the least abusive and most objective course of action on behalf of the child. That course may necessitate considerable effort on behalf of the mother of the child; it will often necessitate taking risks in decision making; it will demand actions which are contrary to many of the prejudicial convictions (see above) which professionals may have once held. If one needs further explanation and justification for the course being advocated here, then one need only consider the outcome of the countless cases in which insufficient support was given to mothers, in which the principal aim and abiding preoccupation was to ensure no risk at all. The most valuable contribution to the welfare principle remains as always: to use it in full recognition of its gravity and complexity, and to cease using it as though it were nothing more than a convenient platitudinous soundbite.

Acknowledging non-abusing mothers

Policy and procedure should clearly differentiate between abusing and non-abusing mothers. Mothers who are unaware of the abuse perpetrated against their children, and who immediately report that abuse when they learn about it, should not be subjected to the rigours and crisis-inducing mechanisms which normally operate in child protection work. A case may be posited suggesting that the mother unwittingly facilitated the abuse (for example, leaving them with unsuitable childminders, dangerous items lying around, etc.) but here again, discretion should be exercised, as such a case is substantially different from that in which a parent deliberately abuses or consciously facilitates another person abusing her child.

Confronting, not reframing domestic violence

Many women approach childcare agencies seeking help because they are routinely subjected to violence by their male partners. Policy and procedure should encourage workers to respect and respond to this request, not compel them to subject the woman to lengthy and intrusive interviewing, attempting to convert it into a child abuse referral (Farmer 1993; McWilliams and McKiernan 1993). It already is a child abuse referral: battering women inescapably harms their children emotionally and psychologically (Jaffe *et al.* 1990; O'Hagan 1993). The prevalence of domestic violence and the frequency with which childcare professionals encounter battered women necessitate policy and procedure based upon a recognition of: (1) the psychology of domestic violence; (2) the multiple abuses (physical, psychological, emotional and social) which the woman endures as a consequence and the adverse impact upon her ability to care adequately for her children; and (3) the emotional and psychological consequences suffered by the child. If children themselves had a voice in the referral and investigative process, their greatest wish would be for workers to rescue their mother from the violence. Policy and procedure, backed up by resources, should offer women an alternative; they should never allow workers the discretion to threaten a woman that her children will be removed (battered women's greatest fear (Hegarty 1993)) if she does not find that alternative herself.

Referrals and anonymous referrals

The frequency with which single parent mothers are subjected to investigative procedures as a consequence of inadequate, malicious, unsubstantiated referrals is a national scandal. Research findings and literature (Besharov 1990; Rickford 1993; Thorpe 1994) on child protection referrals demand fundamental changes in policy and procedure. The problem is primarily a lack of scrutiny in referral taking. The point has already been made – and cannot be made often enough – that the referral-taking task is difficult and complex. It requires tact, confidence and subtlety. It is the foundation upon which rigorous and effective investigative and intervention work is carried out. Policy and procedure should perform two functions: first, to emphasize the foundational aspect of referral-taking and alert workers to the fact that many women-abusing attitudes and practices, whatever their origins, are likely to begin manifesting during this earliest phase of child protection work. Second, comprehensive referral-taking guidelines free of all women-abusing potential should be available, as part of, or incorporated within, procedures. Referral forms need altering. They should contain questions on aspects of the child's welfare (for example, emotional, psychological, social, educational), for which there may be a favourable response, and for which the mother in particular is responsible; in other words, they should not be dominated by a big blank space crying out for details of physical or sexual abuse alone! Sections on male partners and their role and influence need to be inserted. Procedure and policy on *anonymous* referrals need substantial amendment. Staff actually need to be trained for coping with anonymous referrals. No childcare professional belonging to an agency which is part of the child protection network, should be allowed to remain the anonymous source of a child abuse referral (we have found a number of social services departments which do allow childcare professionals to remain anonymous). All childcare professionals are members of the child protection network; this necessitates frankness and honesty between themselves and the principal carers about any concerns they may have.

Avoiding the avoidance of men

Chapter 9 illustrated how policy and procedure facilitate a potent and prevalent form of the abuse of women, namely, the avoidance of men. Previous chapters have demonstrated numerous types of avoidance, how women are abused as a consequence, and how risk to the general health of the child is increased. Perquisite to the necessary modifications in policy and procedure, is policymakers' awareness of the extent of the problem. The wider definition of 'avoidance' provided in Chapter 9 needs to preface whatever guidelines and procedures follow, and childcare workers need to be made aware of the categories of avoidance, and of the frequency of avoidance throughout each phase of childcare work. Here is a reminder of the main categories of avoidance:

- blatant avoidance;
- avoiding men who are present;
- avoiding men by 'defining them out';
- avoiding men by 'trusting mothers';
- avoiding men by relying on grandmothers.

What is required, in effect, is a principle of *non-avoidance of all significant persons* conspicuously placed in the mission statement and/or the statement of philosophy of each childcare agency. This principle needs to be universally acknowledged and endorsed by all childcare professionals. As may be implied in Chapter 9, it would be no easy task adhering to the principle, and there would be numerous obstacles in implementing policies and procedures based upon it. One of those obstacles is professionals' fear of intimidation and violence by men. Fortunately, this obstacle is not so great as it may appear, and erroneous assumptions which have sustained the fears can easily be exposed.

Policy and procedure based upon reality and research

Childcare professionals sometimes avoid men because they believe men pose the greater risk of violence towards them. It is in fact women who are more likely to attack childcare workers. Research demonstrates this convincingly (Rowett 1986; Norris 1991). Childcare workers have little or no contact with men; this lack of contact fuels existing fears of men, giving workers no opportunity to acquire experience and confidence in engaging men, or in realizing why women pose the greater risk; consequently, on the few occasions they do meet men, workers are often apprehensive and predictive of violence. The reason why women pose the greater threat is that they are more frequently and pervasively abused by the childcare system. There are occasions when the abuse is of such intensity and frequency that women are provoked into attack; this is the reason why, contrary to common belief, attacks are likely to come from women who are well known by the workers they attack. They attack out of a *sustained* sense of injustice and not because of some isolated abusive behaviour on the part of the worker. The occasion when childcare workers are more at risk of attack is not, as many believe, during the investigative phase; rather, it is much later, after the intervention phase, when decisions are taken to remove the child, or not to return a child already removed. Here again, the reason for these research-based facts is obvious: the child (or children) is often the one and only source of self-worth and hope for many mothers already burdened by poverty, stigma and isolation. The threat of removal, or a court's approval of a removal which has already taken place (in addition to the humiliations often endured in childcare proceedings), is something that some mothers will not be able to tolerate.

What is written here must not be interpreted as a denial of the fact that men are overwhelmingly the perpetrators of violence, or as a suggestion that childcare workers are never attacked by men, or that the relatively few men they encounter pose no danger to them. On the contrary, male clients have perpetrated many acts of violence against social work childcare workers in particular, and have actually murdered both childcare and mental health workers, in Britain and elsewhere (Norris 1991; Zito 1994). But research findings and the knowledge of experienced childcare workers are important none the less in informing those who formulate the policies and lay down the procedures. Both policy and procedure must expose not just the dangerousness (to both mother and child) of avoiding men, but also the assumption, shared by many inexperienced childcare workers, that women pose no threats to them at all.

Parental participation: policy without rhetoric

The Children Act 1989 is primarily responsible for the current popular usage of terms like 'parental participation', 'partnership', 'cooperation', etc. But as we have seen in Chapters 6 and 8, there are enormous discrepancies both in the interpretation and application of these terms. What must be established at the outset is that women are predominantly the recipients of any degree of participation and partnership: those who do have male partners are still most likely to be the principal focus of attention by childcare agencies; their male partners will have no incentive to be involved; many childcare workers will still want to avoid men, and many men will successfully avoid childcare workers. Single parent mothers are by far the largest category of persons in contact with those agencies, and those responsible for modifying policy and procedure to incorporate principles on parental participation should remain aware of that fact.

Managers and policy makers may believe their childcare policy has taken a significant step towards parental participation by allowing parents to attend part of the case conference, or allowing them to attend only review meetings (three to six months after the initial case conferences). This is not parental participation, nor is it partnership. It is, in fact, worse than allowing no attendance at all, as parents in Thoburn's (1992) research made clear. All 20 parents in O'Hagan's (1994) research expressed a strong desire to attend the whole conference. If managers cannot embrace this spirit of partnership and participation with adequate policy, they should state so, unambiguously. They should not, through flourishing rhetoric, attempt to convey the impression that their's *is* a policy that articulates and promotes parental participation when most convincingly it is not. Parents, particularly lone single parent mothers, have to be prepared and supported throughout the formidable task of attending case conferences. Reference has been made (see Chapter 8) to the irony of millions of pounds being spent preparing professionals for parental attendance, and no resources whatsoever being spent on preparing those who need preparation and support far more, that is, the parents themselves.

Case conferences have been an easy option for childcare agencies, upon which to experiment with parental participation (and not very taxing for those modifying their existing policy). There is ample evidence, in the many research projects referred to throughout this text, to suggest that even in this very narrow focal point in child protection work, agencies are falling far short of minimum expectations (for example, 59 per cent of parents who attended case conferences in Farmer's (1993) research found the experience intimidating, embarrassing and humiliating). But what of the other phases of childcare work? How is 'parental participation' being implemented during the crisis-laden referral, investigation and intervention phases? The fact is that many managers have not even begun to think of parental participation during these phases; consequently, they are in no position to define it, nor to formulate policy and procedure to promote it. Parental participation is a principle which should pervade the whole process of child protection and childcare work.

Conclusion

Childcare systems are necessary, but they do not have to be abusive. Abuses may continue to be perpetrated against mothers as a consequence of root and branch changes in the organization and structure of childcare systems, but many other features of those systems can be improved dramatically; their vulnerability to the political climate of the day, for example. Frontline professionals need to be politically conscious; they need to be acutely sensitive to the shifting tides of public opinions and prejudices often moulded by politicians, and the impact these may have upon their clients generally. Single parent mothers are particularly vulnerable in this respect and professionals can ensure, through vigilance and rigorous scrutiny, that they do not become a mere instrument of political and public whim hostile to single parents or other groups. The 1989 Children Act needs some amendments. A number of sections allow local authorities too much discretion which can easily result in the abuse of parents. The Act's innovative and welcome promotion of the policy aimed at getting suspected abusers removed, has been misinterpreted and exploited in pursuit of a thoroughly improper practice of threatening mothers with the removal of the child. There is an urgent need to expose and prohibit such practice. Mothers generally, and poor, inarticulate, single parent mothers in particular, stand to lose out in the present controversy surrounding the Child Support Agency. They may become the target of even greater interrogation and intrusion by CSA investigators, whose activities in respect of fathers are likely to be seriously curtailed. The enactment of potentially abusive legislation often follows crusades and campaigns; the substantial changes demanded by anti-CSA campaigners may result in legislation which undermines the principle of fathers being responsible for their children. Another example of potentially abusive legislation is the repeal of the Homeless Person's Act, which comes in the wake of a sometimes virulent campaign directed against single parent mothers. Many of these mothers will be the principal victims of the repeal, and childcare workers must systematically record and report its consequences on the welfare of children. It is quite possible for childcare workers, as it has been for many other groups of workers, to contest abusive legislation which has its origins in an abusive climate of opinion.

Inappropriate motivating factors may cause professionals to abuse mothers. Motivation should be subject to regular self-scrutiny on the part of the professional, and constant monitoring within the supervisory process. Policy and procedures in childcare agencies need thorough scrutiny, particularly on the following: the application of the welfare principle; attitude to non-abusing mothers; responses to mothers subjected to domestic violence; inadequate referral taking; malicious anonymous referrals about single parent mothers; the wholesale avoidance of men in childcare work; and, the implementation of parental participation. These are all subject areas necessitating modification (and sometimes substantial change) in existing policies and procedures. Policy and procedure are the most influential core components of all childcare systems. Those who are now formulating them have the opportunity to eradicate many of the abuses of women which their predecessors have unwittingly facilitated.

12

Implications for trainers

Introduction

The contents of previous chapters have implications for all childcare professionals, and those responsible for formulating, enacting and implementing childcare law, policy and procedures. This chapter, however, will concentrate on the implications for *the trainers* of childcare workers. This is for two reasons: first, trainers are crucial in any strategy which aims to confront the abuse of women; and second, the issue of training as a contributory or preventive factor in the abuse of women, has not been tackled before. The contents of this chapter are relevant to all levels of childcare training. 'Gender' and 'anti-discriminatory practice' are now prominent components in most childcare courses, yet many students leave courses no more able to avoid abusing women than when their training commenced. How can trainers and training establishments best prepare workers for withstanding the multiple women-abusing influences which, as preceding chapters have demonstrated, are in abundance in childcare agencies? Since agencies are now significant partners in training, the need to tackle the matter is more urgent than ever. Self-awareness is crucial in this matter, as is the teaching of theory and the preparation for practice in many of the potentially abusive situations previously described (particularly in Chapter 8). This chapter will provide some simple basic models for enhancing self-awareness, teaching relevant theory, and engaging, rather than avoiding, men.

Training for the prevention of the abuse of women

Self-awareness

How can the abuse of women occur in childcare to the extent that it does, when anti-discriminatory policy has been such a major preoccupation for course tutors and practice teachers alike? One certain reason is that child-care students have not been given the opportunity of exploring the potential for abuse which exists within each and everyone of us. If this painful self-exploration did occur, then students, their course tutors and their practice teachers, would have to acknowledge the extent of the problem, which in turn, would be an incentive for strategies in training and management to cope with it. Whatever has been said about the origins of abuse against women within childcare systems, in laws, theories, policies and procedures, that abuse is, ultimately, the result of actions by individuals within those systems. In Chapter 2, we stressed that it is unlikely that childcare workers are always aware of the fact that they are abusing women; the crisis nature of much of childcare work, and constant pressure revolving around their statutory duty to minimize risk, does not afford them the luxury of calm reflection during their interventions. A major responsibility in training, therefore, is to make childcare workers of the future aware of their potential to abuse.

The challenge of self-awareness

There are risks in this self-exploration. Trainers seek to inspire students. They make every effort to sustain the enthusiasm and idealism with which students enrolled on courses. They aim to give the student confidence and enable him/her to acquire the competence to provide quality service to clients; in short, they strive to enable students to feel good about themselves. Making students look into their souls in order to find something potentially nasty has never been a part of training and recruitment in childcare programmes. But increasingly trainers in numerous professions are realizing the necessity for students to explore their vulnerabilities and to learn of their capacity for poor quality service delivered through discriminatory practice, and to learn about those situations of crises and conflict and danger, in which good quality anti-discriminatory practice may be forsaken. Trainers have to facilitate students contemplating the possibility of themselves as abusers, and to identify: (1) aspects of their own character, style and personality; (2) events in their own past lives, and (3) convictions and prejudices they have acquired, etc., any of which may be conducive to the abuse of women. As Kirwan (1994) states:

> egalitarian social work is not possible without a proper understanding of the wider gender issues which impinge on the relationship with the

client. As part of this understanding, personal attitudes and biases of social workers have to be confronted. Training is one of the most appropriate places in which to tackle this personal development and change. (p. 142)

Kirwan acknowledges how difficult it is for training staff to explore gender honestly and rigorously, when the composition and hierarchy of training establishments mirror the imbalance of power and influence in a patriarchal society which they serve. This does not only apply to teaching gender; for example, in Northern Ireland, where agencies and training establishments are preoccupied with combating sectarianism in the workplace, social work trainers have difficulty in exploring, openly and honestly, even among themselves, their own contribution to the sectarian divide. No doubt the same applies to those training establishments preoccupied with teaching about racism.

Tutors and practice teachers: a partnership for training

The starting point, therefore, is within trainers themselves – that is, course tutors and practice teachers – within the partnership of training. This partnership concept is important. It would be tempting to believe that since childcare agencies abuse women so routinely, then practice teachers based in those agencies have little contribution to make in training students not to abuse. Practice teachers are vitally necessary in combating the abuse. They are acutely aware of the potential for abuse within their agencies; they will recall complex and risk-laden situations in which decisions made and actions taken, in good faith, seemingly with sound judgement, nevertheless ended up being abusive. Indeed, some of the contents of these chapters are actually based upon the experiences of practice teachers. The significant role which practice teachers can play helps determine the timing of self-awareness training. The nature of the challenge it presents to students is such that it should not be attempted until the latter part of the course; it should, ideally, take place after the student has had at least one placement and before the final placement. Whatever the timing, however, the training should always be jointly planned and implemented by college based tutors and agency based practitioners.

What about the other half of the partnership? The vast majority of tutors, based in academic training establishments, were once practitioners themselves. They will have no difficulty remembering how they, too, once belonged to abusive childcare systems. They will understand, as Milner (1993) quickly understood when she returned to practice, how easy it is to abuse women, and how difficult it is to resist all of the multiple abusive influences and processes within childcare systems. This is not to advocate some kind of catharsis or confessional for trainers; it is merely to suggest that this acknowledgement and understanding will increase confidence in enabling their childcare students to do likewise.

The mechanics and processes of joint training on self-awareness can be worked out by individual partnerships. The eventual implementation of the training will necessitate providing exercises and frameworks to enable students to explore the potential for abuse within themselves. The frameworks in previous chapters may help. Each of the components of abusive childcare systems, can be used to generate a series of questions for the student. The exercise may be enhanced with the help of actual cases (many of the cases in previous chapters would do). One important and non-negotiable condition is that exercises in self-awareness on this topic should *not* be done in group discussions; nothing is better calculated to ensure inhibition, and a lack of the honesty and rigour which the exercise necessitates; alternatively, students may reveal some past experience of great intimacy, and therefore feel immensely vulnerable; too late then (a lesson painfully learnt in training on child sexual abuse). These exercises may be carried out between student, practice teacher and tutor, or between student and tutor only, and the results later shared fully with the practice teacher. In either case, the results must be treated in the strictest confidence.

Let us now consider some sample questions that might usefully be asked. The following sections begin with general questions and progress to the particular. The latter should provide the opportunity for more focused and more challenging self-exploration. Students will have to be reassured about the outcome of this exercise: they may have difficulty in answering some of the questions (very understandable); or they may think some of their answers jeopardize their prospects of completing the course. On the contrary – as Kirwan (1994) implies – the realization and acknowledgement of the potential for abuse of women should be stressed as a major and necessary leap forward in professional development.

Prevailing political climate

1 What are my views and feelings on women's issues (or issues which seriously impact upon women) which have become the topic of political debate? For example, on:

- single parent mothers;
- Child Support Agency;
- adoption/transracial adoption;
- repeal of the Homeless Person's Act;
- child sexual abuse;
- *in vitro* fertilization;
- abortion, etc.

2 What is the origin of my views and feelings on these issues?

3 Could any of these views and feelings lead to discriminatory practice against women? Illustrate with a particular case.

The welfare of the child is paramount

1 What is my understanding of this principle and its operation in childcare work?
2 What are my thoughts and feelings on the relationship between the welfare of the child and the rights of parents?
3 In what types of situation am I likely to take action which I believe is in the interests of the welfare of the child, yet is very much contrary to the parents' wishes?
4 What personal experiences in childhood or adolescence, and in my family life generally, are likely to influence my thoughts and feelings on these two concepts: the welfare of the child and the rights of the parents?
5 Could any of my thoughts and feelings on this issue lead me to actions which may be abusive to the mother of a child?

Common beliefs

1 List some common beliefs about women in general, and about mothers who are clients of childcare workers in particular. Do I share any of those beliefs? For example, do I believe:

  ● that most mothers of children abused by male partners, collude in the abuse?
  ● that mothers always cope?
  ● that grandmothers always know best?
  ● that male partners of mothers are not worth bothering about?

2 Where do my beliefs on women generally, and mothers in particular, originate? – a particular culture? community? educational system? family? literature?
3 Which beliefs may influence my practice? And how? (give examples)
4 In what childcare situations may any of these common beliefs cause me to abuse, or contribute to my abusing, women? Think through such a situation and describe in detail.

Race

1 What do I know about mothers of ethnic groups with whom I may work?
2 What are my views and feelings on transracial fostering and adoption? And on different child-rearing practices which I am aware of?
3 What is the difference between fact and knowledge about mothers from different ethnic groups, and stereotype?
4 What negative stereotype of the mothers of ethnic groups am I aware of?
5 Do I share any negative stereotypes mentioned above?
6 How does negative stereotype affect practice?

Women with disability
1 What are my views and feelings on particular disabilities – for example, cerebral palsy? multiple sclerosis? alcoholism? mental illness? limblessness (caused by thalidomide, an accident, etc.) blindness? deafness? learning difficulties?
2 How do any of these disabilities impact upon the quality of care a mother may provide?
3 Should any of these disabilities preclude the right of the disabled woman to have and to be the main carer of a child?
4 Can I envisage a situation in which I feel very strongly that a mother's disability and her environment should compel me and my agency to ensure her child is removed.

Working style, personality, and character In many of the case scenarios in previous chapters, the workers exhibited distinct characteristics and styles of working which contributed to and increased the sense of injustice and abuse endured by the mother. The following questions require students to focus on their own style and emotional interaction between themselves and mothers during differing phases of work.

1 Recalling a child abuse investigation which I may have carried out, or imagining one that I might carry out in the future, how would I describe my approach, attitude and feelings to the mother of the child? Am I likely to be highly sensitive and sympathetic, tense, secretive, determined, open and honest, arrogant, confident, tactful, direct, formal, informal, etc.? (Apply the same type of question to other case scenarios structured around other phases of childcare work – for example, intervention, care proceedings, etc.)
2 Could I imagine myself participating in a dawn raid to remove children? Could I become totally preoccupied with the welfare of the child and ignore the feelings of the mother of the child?
3 Could I bring undue pressure (that is, subtle and not-so-subtle threats) to bear upon the mother to get her male partner removed? How might I feel if I was asked to facilitate secret videoing of a mother who was suspected of harming her child?
4 If, during an investigation, it feels as though a mother is successfully resisting the process of investigation (that is, denying abuse, refusing to answer questions, showing anger, cursing, swearing, etc.), what impact is this likely to have on my attitude and actions towards that mother?

Self-awareness on avoidance strategies
1 In what situations do I avoid contact with men? Explain why.
2 In which particular phase of childcare work am I most reluctant to have contact with men. Explain why.

3 What strategies am I likely to adopt to avoid men during the phases identified above?
4 What are the possible consequences of my avoidance for: (1) the mother of the child? (2) the child?

Outcome

The outcome of this self-exploration exercise will be shared by tutor and practice teacher. It is merely a beginning exercise which should lead to further exploration. On the basis of what the student reveals in these exercises, the tutor and practice teacher have the responsibility of prioritizing the student's various potentials for abusing women, and matching these with potentially abusive features of the placement (or potentially abusive features of the local childcare scene generally), in which such potential is likely to be realized. For example, a student may make it abundantly clear that he/she believes race is unimportant in fostering and adoption. The policy of the department may be similar; the law certainly is moving in that direction; the local press may have racist views on the matter; the area of the placement may be one in which there are a high number of black children placed for adoption and fostering. Given all these factors, the student's abuse of black, natural mothers in fostering and adoption cases is not just likely; it is inevitable. Similarly, a student may disclose that she has great difficulty in any kind of contact with men because she endured years of abuse by her father, and witnessed him abusing her mother throughout her childhood. The location of the placement may have a high incidence of childcare problems caused by, or greatly exacerbated by, domestic violence. In the absence of careful monitoring, there is a strong likelihood of this student avoiding men, abusing women and heightening risk to children.

What then has to be done when students have completed this exercise. Take that last student for example. It is highly likely that she will be totally unaware of the abusive potential of avoiding men. The contents of these chapters, research literature and child abuse enquiry reports should easily convince her otherwise. But she needs a lot more. She may need additional highly focused tutorials and supervision sessions. She is *not* an untypical student. Black *et al.*'s (1993) research clearly indicates the high number of students on welfare courses who have had seriously problematic pasts. They recommend that training should: 'incorporate into the curriculum approaches to sensitize students to the need to recognize the potential impact of their own personal psychosocial background on the helping process' (p. 179). More specifically, this student will additionally need training that gives her confidence and competence in engaging male clients. And, whatever changes are being sought in her attitude and approach, they need to be underpinned by a firm theoretical base. In the next section we will explore some of the implications for teaching a non-discriminatory theory.

Teaching theory: implications for trainers

Childcare theory has become an important part in the training of childcare workers. In Chapter 10 we outlined the behaviour analytic approach which, we believe, has the potential to prevent the abuse of women in childcare work. Teaching behaviour analytic theory to childcare workers has a number of implications for trainers. First, childcare trainers have to be familiar with the theory themselves. Behavioural theory is not new to childcare training (McAuley 1981); however, it is often misunderstood, misapplied and misrepresented. Childcare trainers who endeavour to teach this approach, therefore, must understand and represent the theory correctly (Nye (1992) offers comprehensive clarification). Second, behaviour analysis is constantly developing. New knowledge is gained through experimentation or applied research. New knowledge has to be integrated into existing frameworks. In order to teach childcare students comprehensively, childcare trainers must keep abreast of the latest developments. Third, childcare trainers who are taking the challenge seriously of developing and teaching behaviour analysis in childcare work must be at the forefront of related research. The importance of protecting women and integrating men into childcare work has been emphasized throughout this book. There is a lack of research in this area that can only be filled by committed childcare researchers and trainers. Fourth, childcare trainers who are committed to teaching non-abusive theory must find teaching methods that are effective, enjoyable and stimulating for students. They must develop training methods that are innovative and challenging (Jason1984; Keenan1993). We have suggested some ideas of how attitudes and beliefs can be challenged and how awareness of the abuse of women can be raised in the previous section of this chapter. We will now introduce some ideas of how theory can be taught effectively to prevent the abuse of women in childcare work.

Using theory to teach theory

The following programme assignment schedule is an example of how behaviour analysis can be taught to childcare students who are aware of the potential for abusive childcare practices. Behaviour analysis is based on basic principles or laws of behaviour. These principles are in operation when behaviour changes and develops. Behaviour analysis can be used effectively in the protection of women clients because the behaviour of women clients and workers is analysed according to these principles. Hypothetical guesses about internal causes are avoided. It makes sense to utilize our knowledge about the basic principles of behaviour when training childcare students to use behaviour analysis to prevent the abuse of women in childcare work (Michael, 1993). In a sense, theory is used to teach the theory.

Assignment schedule

The assignment for the course is three-fold.
Part A of the assignment is a multiple choice test. This test is based on teaching during the college block and home study. The test is held on three occasions. The best result counts towards the overall grade.
Part B is a report of a behaviour change project in which students are required to apply *the new childcare theory to a case from their placement*. Guidelines are provided in Sulzer-Azaroff and Reese (1982).
Part C: Each student presents their project to their tutorial group. The presentations last approximately 20 minutes and follow general presentation guidelines provided to the students.
Grading is compensatory. Part A counts 25%, Part B counts 60%, and Part C counts 15% towards the overall final grade.

The assignment schedule is based on the principle of 'shaping'. Step-by-step, students are taught theory and non-abusive practice towards women clients. First, students are taught basic theory by lectures, videos, role plays and discussion groups. The assignment for this early part of the course (Part A) is a multiple choice test that was applied on three occasions. The best result counted towards the overall mark. The effect of repeated feedback and reinforcement was that students' performance improved. Figure 12.1 illustrates the progress made by a group of childcare students.

The test results show that students were becoming increasingly familiar with the basics of behavioural theory. They could now begin to apply theory to practice. Part B of the assignment, therefore, required students to conduct a project in which they had to apply effectively principles of behaviour with a client during placement. Students' awareness of the potential of abuse in practice was integrated into the theoretical framework. Guidelines on how to conduct this kind of project are provided by Sulzer-Azaroff and Reese (1982).

Two examples of student projects will serve to illustrate the usefulness of carefully arranged assignment schedules for student learning and for the application of non-abusive childcare theory.

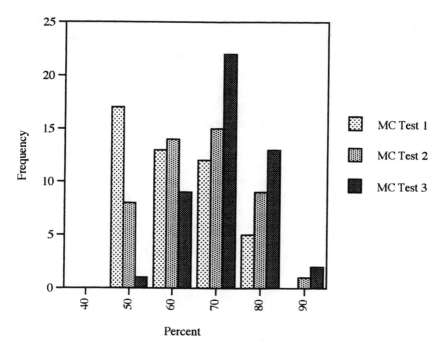

Figure 12.1 Multiple choice test results

Student G. was on placement in a refuge for women who had experienced domestic violence. The potential for abuse of these women by childcare workers is vast. Children in refuges often cause concern and mothers are the only carer available for investigation and intervention. The student was asked to act as key worker for a newly admitted mother and her 19 month old baby son. There was serious concern about the welfare of the boy. Apart from some health related problems his behaviour did not seem that of a child of his age. He usually sat on a chair in the living room by himself. He did not show much interest in his mother and remained seemingly unmoved when she came to lift him. He also could not walk. Rather than write an essay about the stages of development and a discussion on avoidant attachment (which is the traditional method of student assessment) and thereby unintentionally blaming and abusing the boy's mother, the student had to do a project in behaviour analysis for her assignment. She began her project by identifying 'walking' as the behaviour to deal with first. She carefully observed context and consequences of the boy's walking behaviour. She found that none of his attempts to walk were reinforced. She explained this to the boy's mother and together they devised a programme in which they reinforced the boy for attempts at walking. The boy learnt to walk relatively quickly. The response from the mother was not surprising. She took great interest in her son's achievements and soon taught him all sorts of other behaviours. The concerns about the boy's welfare diminished and the mother was not abused in the process. On the contrary, she was respected, involved and in charge.

Another example of application of non-abusive childcare theory was the project of student O.

> Student O. was on placement in a family and childcare field work office. The case he used for his project involved a single mother and her two sons, aged six and eight. There was serious concern about the welfare of the boys. They seemed largely out of their mother's control and on one occasion the mother had bruised one of them when she grabbed his arm, trying to restrain him. The boys were continuously fighting and arguing and the mother was worried that one day she would seriously harm them. Student O. analysed the context and the consequences of the boys' fighting behaviour and identified the reinforcement involved. He and the mother planned a programme in which they would use contingent reinforcement for peaceful play and cooperation between the boys. The boys' behaviour soon improved. This case has serious potential for mother blaming and abuse by childcare workers, or care orders for the boys. The approach taken by the student enabled the mother actively to achieve behavioural change in her boys. She felt proud of her achievement and the concern about the level of physical punishment was reduced.

The student had put theory into practice effectively (see Jason (1984) for further examples of student projects).

In part C of the assignment students reported their project to each other in their tutorial groups. This presentation took place immediately after the students returned from placement. Presenting their projects enabled students to learn from each other (modelling) and to give each other direct feedback on their performance.

Holland (1978) summed up the benefits of behaviour analysis for childcare practice and training when he said that:

> the standard use of victim-blaming and inner causes itself has a be-havioural basis, in that it reinforces the status quo; this is so even though the science of behaviour has made such inner causes unsatis-factory as explanations of behaviour. A wider dissemination of the methods for analyzing controlling contingencies can accelerate the creation of a non-oppressive society and the passing away of the social problems for which victims are themselves so often blamed. (p. 37)

The above assignment schedule was an example of how this can be achieved with childcare students.

Training to avoid avoiding men

Avoiding men is one of the most prevalent and effective means by which women are abused within childcare systems. The determination not to avoid men should be a core principle in the mission statements of both agencies and childcare training establishments. Trainers and practice teachers in the various childcare professions, particularly social work and health visiting, may recall how ill-prepared and untrained they were for engaging men when they left their own courses as qualified professionals. That experience, and awareness of the consequences of avoiding men, should be an effective motivating force in ensuring that the childcare professionals of the future will not be similarly handicapped. Chapter 10 provided a theoretical base challenging any tendency in practice to avoid men; Chapter 11 suggested necessary changes in policies and procedures which facilitate avoidance. The remainder of this chapter will concentrate on some specific training tasks.

Structure of training on how not to avoid

The knowledge base A basic structure of training on avoidance can be elicited from the contents of Chapter 9. Students should be able to:

1 Define 'avoidance' in its widest sense.
2 Accept that avoidance takes place throughout each of the seven phases of child protection and childcare work – that is, referral, investigation, intervention, case conference, care proceedings, fostering and adoption.
3 Understand and provide examples of the differing categories of avoidance – for example, blatant, 'defining men out', etc.
4 Provide many examples of these types of avoidance, in real or imagined cases.
5 Understand and explain how each type of avoidance of men can *lead to various types of abuse of women* in each phase of childcare work.
6 Give numerous examples of any of the above abuses in real or imagined cases.
7 Understand and explain how the avoidance of men can heighten risk to the child.
8 Suggest and explain various motivations of workers avoiding men.
9 Recall how the avoidance of men was a persistent feature of nearly all the child abuse enquiry reports, and to know the details of those cases in which avoidance proved disastrous for the child (for example, Tyra Henry, Kimberly Carlile, Toni Dales, etc.).
10 Quote research evidence on violence against workers.

Identifying and prioritizing core skills

Practice teachers and tutors are well aware from their own experiences of situations in which avoidance is likely, and what precisely is the major obstacle preventing workers from avoiding. For example, men perceived as violent, inability to communicate with men, believing men unimportant, etc. The responses of students to the self-awareness exercise – especially the section on avoidance – will also help in initiating a programme enabling students to acquire skills, attitude and approach, deemed to be the most necessary. Parts of that programme require little effort and challenge to either student or trainers; for example, dealing with the first phase of work: referral taking.

Referrals It is very easy to explore the extent of the inclination to avoid men, or questions about men, in referral taking; and if the extent is considerable, it is just as easy to encourage students to formulate a comprehensive and effective set of guidelines ensuring non-avoiding inclinations. But this needs to be tested. It can be tested on placement (and should be), but, it can also be tested in the college setting. Student volunteers can be invited to take referrals alone in one of the college offices. The referrer, *unknown to the student,* may be a colleague or friend, phoning in from outside. These 'referrers' must be carefully primed to give referrals which are totally lacking in any information about males who are probably significant to the child. Before the appointed time, the class discuss all the possibilities; when the student returns, his or her experiences are shared with the class. Detailed written feedback from the referrer is provided later. It is a challenging, productive and often humorous exercise.

Investigation and intervention Role play is a useful tool for practising non-avoidance during the investigative and intervention phase. Without careful preparation and discipline, however, this particular kind of role play can easily degenerate into farce, with some players ending up humiliated and turned off role play for ever, and trainers and teachers alike concluding that it was a futile exercise not to be repeated. Role plays have to be carefully constructed if the goal is to be achieved; the audience members have to realize the crucial role they can play, for good or ill. The basic goal is to offer students contrasting situations which accentuate the difference of challenge posed by the *presence* and *absence* of men. Let the investigating worker (a student volunteer) experience a possibly frightened woman opening the door at a time when nobody else is at home. Dead easy! Then let them experience a tough, questioning woman staring distrustfully and angrily at them backed up by a six foot gangsterish looking male towering over her from behind (this sounds like a stereotype, but the scenario and impact upon the worker, are common). Let them walk into the room in which a mother and her children are present; then walk in when there is also an aggressive looking male partner sprawled over the sofa and the television is blaring; let the students engage in these contrasting scenarios numerous times, sharing their thoughts, feelings, and challenge as they do. They will reveal a host of reasons for the difficulty they are experiencing. The observing students will share what they feel is most difficult for them. One of the main reasons for the difficulty is the sheer unfamiliarity of the experience; students simply have never been in this predicament before: facing a man in a child abuse investigation. What may also emerge is the realization that the anticipation of aggression or violence *from the man* is exacerbating the student's difficulty, thus greatly undermining their confidence to be able to explain who they are and why they are there. This is where research and the work experience of tutors and practice teachers proves invaluable. The period of initial contact between investigative worker and suspected abusers really is the least potentially violent phase of childcare work (apart from the referral phase). Role play enables students not only to play out this anticipation of violence, but, more importantly, to explore the experience and perception of the man whose presence is provoking this fear. Students will very quickly learn just how unlikely it is for a man to attack a government officer who he has met for the first time, who is merely doing his/her duty of investigating a child abuse referral. Men in this situation, even (or particularly) men with a record of violence, or convictions for violence, retain a very healthy awareness of the consequences of such an attack. It is very important for trainers to expose the myth that workers are likely to be attacked by men during investigation. However, it is equally important to alert and to prepare students for the high incidence of attack by mothers in the later phases of childcare work (Rowett 1986; Norris 1991).

Too much concentration on the potential for violence is unnecessary. Far more likely is the man's and woman's reluctant cooperation. There is still the enormous potential for avoidance of the man. Students can be invited to suggest appropriate and inappropriate reaching out and engaging the man as the investigation proceeds. A consensus will emerge on what is appropriate and inappropriate; it is usually right, though be prepared for the occasional suggestion, that is utterly wrong: for example, 'can I speak to you alone in another room, Mrs Smith [*about this partner of yours whom we believe is abusing your kids!*]'.

Seeking authenticity

The student may now be thoroughly familiar with all aspects of knowledge on avoidance; they may have learnt a great deal about their inclination for avoiding men in the self-awareness and role play exercises; they may indeed be a lot more confident. It will be immensely helpful now if some of them can have the opportunity to do an investigative visit to an actual home and family, in which a male is present. One needs very accommodating friends for this exercise (the college's drama department is never short of members willing to play the roles of parents in their own homes); but, provided one prepares well, the benefits are enormous. Students may initially resist the idea, but, when those who volunteer return and share their experiences with the class, the majority of students are likely to demand the same opportunity!

Similar types of exercises and role plays can reveal situations in which students are tempted to avoid men throughout each phase of childcare work. The cumulative effects of self-awareness, a comprehensive knowledge base, and the opportunity to observe and advise one's student colleagues as they embark upon *non-avoiding* practice in role play, are three-fold: first, the student's awareness and familiarity with the problem of avoidance is greatly enhanced. Second, they can identify what aspect of male presence causes them difficulty; consequently, their confidence in dealing with the difficulty is substantially increased. Third, they then have ample opportunity, in group discussion, additional role play, placement supervision, tutorials, and written assignments, to formulate strategies maximizing their potential for engaging men.

Such exercises, of course, offer many additional training opportunities. The presence of a man, for example, does not only raise the problem of how to engage *him*, but it also sheds some light on the student's awareness of the impact of gender, and on his/her capacities with groups in particular; on the latter for example, how to engage more than one person; where to position oneself; how to prevent one person dominating, maintaining the other's interest, etc.

Students cannot be expected to be able to carry out comprehensive and successful child abuse investigations at the point at which they qualify, and it should be made clear to them that that is not the purpose of any of the above exercises. But it is imperative none the less, that throughout their professional training, in both college and practice locations, they be given every possible opportunity to meet the challenge of avoidance, which is such a major contributory factor towards the abuse of women in childcare work. The sooner the prevention of avoiding men becomes a compulsory and tested objective on every childcare course (however it may be achieved) the better.

Conclusion

Trainers on childcare qualifying courses, and practice teachers on placement, can make a major contribution towards reducing the amount of abuse perpetrated against women in childcare work. This chapter has suggested what that contribution may be in three distinct phases of training: first, training in self-awareness – that is, students being given the opportunity to explore their own potential for abusing women and the origins of that potential; second, teaching theory significantly different from many of the potentially abusive child developmental theories traditionally and predominantly taught; and third, enabling students to overcome the pervasive and endemic problem of avoiding men in childcare work. This is merely a beginning. After training, professionally qualified workers themselves can continue intensifying their resolve not to abuse women, either wittingly or unwittingly; and they can also become increasingly vigilant in preventing themselves from becoming merely the tools of abusive childcare systems.

Epilogue

A few months ago, a lecturer was coming to the end of the three-week family and childcare sequence in the Diploma in Social Work course. The sequence had revolved around the case of a single parent mother who had two young children. She worked in the evening to supplement her welfare entitlements. She cohabited with a man who looked after the children while she worked. One evening, the man battered one of the children. Neighbours heard the screams and reported it. Social services were called; the police were involved.

This is a very brief outline of a case which was described to the students in detail (not unlike the case at the beginning of Chapter 8) and which provided valuable material for discussion on the ethical, legal, gender and practice implications. Throughout the three-week sequence, the lecturer and his colleagues, including colleagues in childcare agencies, frequently highlighted the potential for abusing the woman in this case. Students were very interested, and gave every indication that they were aware of that potential.

In role play, however, some of the students perceived the woman very negatively. They were given some suggestions and boundaries for playing particular roles, but they often stepped beyond those boundaries, and used their imaginations rather more, and rather more negatively, than had been anticipated. The positive and negative perceptions did not divide easily along particular stereotypes of professional roles; for example, it might have been assumed that social workers would express positive, sensitive and sympathetic views of the woman, and police and/or teachers would express harsh, critical comments about her. On the contrary, the social worker and team leader who had decided that the children should be taken into care, were highly critical of the woman.

Some allowance may be made for these views in the fact that the students were role playing, that they had designated roles, and that they were given the responsibility of convincing others (including the audience) that removal was the best thing. Indeed, in discussion after the role play, students readily acknowledged that perhaps they had gone over the top in their criticism of the mother. However, in the written assignment handed in six weeks later, the lecturer was surprised to find some of those criticisms reoccurring. One student in fact prefaced her assignment with a very clear statement about this mother's responsibility for the abuse and neglect of her children.

There are numerous interpretations which one might make of this event. For example, the teaching on the abuse of women may not have been very effective; or that students had been greatly influenced by their practice placements from which they may have emerged with unshakeable convictions that children should be rescued from abuse at all costs; or, that insufficient preparation had been given to the role play, and that a competitive edge had crept in (as it nearly always does in role play), making some students preoccupied with impressing the audience by winning the argument, rather than getting inside the heads of the professionals they were playing, and seeing things more clearly (that possibility however would not explain some of the statements in the written assignments which were submitted a long time after the role play). Perhaps these were contributory factors, but they do not provide the whole answer.

The *cause* of the abuse of women is not the insensitivity of individual childcare workers, nor can the eradication of the abuse of women be achieved by any individual trainer or childcare manager. What the students demonstrated was the profound nature of the problem of the abuse of women, and that whatever efforts are made by individual trainers, managers, and, indeed, childcare workers, to do something about it, the obstacle to success will remain formidable. Awareness, sensitivity, idealism, enthusiasm and goodness – all those qualities we witness daily in childcare students – simply were not enough to resist covert and overt abusing forces which emerged throughout the role play exercises, and beyond. This experience is not unique; it is precisely the same experience of someone far more knowledgeable then any of those students, namely, Milner (1993) whose work has been a source of inspiration and motivation to us. As a committed feminist, a woman, a trainer, a practitioner, Milner returned from training to practice only to find herself and her child protection colleagues overwhelmed by an abusive childcare system, and herself becoming an unwilling participant in the more covert manifestations of abuse. Yet, in honesty, hope lies.

The abuse of women is not inevitable. We could have demonstrated this point by many examples, from our own experiences as practitioners, from the experiences of our colleagues, and from the reports of practice teachers supervising students (no doubt Milner could have done the same). But space is limited, and time is marching on, and we believe the substantial space and time we have given to the analysis of the abuse of women, the identification of how that abuse manifests itself, and, consequences for both women and their children, was justified. We approached the task of writing this book knowing that there was more than adequate evidence of the abuse of women in childcare; little did we know that evidence would increase significantly by the time we had finished. We hope that the final section of the book, charting different courses in law, policy and procedure, in childcare theory, and in the training of childcare workers, is a reasonable basis upon which to formulate an effective non-discriminatory practice in childcare work. We hope this effort on our part, is merely a little step towards the destination of respect for all.

References

Aldgate, J. (1991) Attachment theory and its application to child care social work: an introduction, in J. Lishman (ed.) *Handbook of Theory for Practice Teachers in Social Work*. London: Jessica Kingsley.

Atkinson, R.L., Atkinson, R.C. and Hilgard, E.R. (1983) *Introduction to Psychology*, 8th edn. New York: Harcourt Brace Jovanovich.

Baer, D.M. (1970) An age-irrelevant concept of development. *Journal of Developmental Psychology, Merrill-Palmer Quarterly*, 16: 238–45.

Baer, D.M. (1973) The control of developmental process: Why wait? in J.R. Nesselroade and H.W. Reese (eds) *Lifespan Developmental Psychology*. New York, London: Academic Press.

Baer, D.M., Peterson, R.F. and Sherman, J.A. (1967) Developing imitation by reinforcing behavioral similarity to a model. *Journal of the Experimental Analysis of Behavior*, 10: 405–16.

Baldwin, J.D. and Baldwin, J.I. (1986) *Behavior Principles in Everday Life*. London: Prentice-Hall.

Barnes, M. and Maple, N. (1992) *Women and Mental Health: Challenging the Stereotype*. Birmingham: Venture.

Barrett, M. (1988) *Women's Oppression Today*. New York, London: Verso.

Baum, W.M. (1994) *Understanding Behaviorism. Science, Behavior and Culture*. New York: Harper Collins.

BBC1 (1993) *Panorama*, 20 September.

BBC1 (1994) *Panorama*, 16 May.

BBC2 (1992) *Screenplay: 'Bad Girl'*, 15 July.

BBC2 (1994a) *Horizon*, 31 January.

BBC2 (1994b) *Newsnight*, 13 July.

Beale, J. (1986) *Women in Ireland. Voices of Change*. London: Macmillan.

Beck, A.T. (1976) *Cognitive Therapy and the Emotional Disorders*. New York: International University Press.

Beck, J.G. and Barlow, D.H. (1984) Unraveling the nature of sex roles, in E.A. Blechman (ed.) *Behavior Modification with Women*. New York, London: The Guilford Press.

Bell, M. (1993) See no evil, speak no evil, hear no evil. *Community Care*, 28 October: 2–3.

Belotti, E.G. (1975) *Little Girls. Social Conditioning and Its Effects on the Stereotyped Role of Women during Infancy*. London: Writers and Readers.

Benedict, M., Zuravin, S., Brandt, D. and Abbey, H. (1994) Types and frequency of child maltreatment by family foster care providers in an urban population. *Child Abuse and Neglect*, 18(7): 577–85.

Besharov, D. (1990) *Recognising Child Abuse: A Guide for the Concerned*. Washington: Free Press.

Bexley (1982) *Report of the Panel of Enquiry*. London Borough of Bexley: Bexley Area Health Authority.

Bijou, S.W. (1993) *Behavior Analysis of Child Development*. Reno: Context Press.

Black, P.N., Jeffreys, D. and Hartley, E.K. (1993) Personal history of psychosocial trauma in the early life of social work and business students. *Journal of Social Work Education*, 29(2): 171–80.

Black, R. (1992) *Orkney: A Place of Safety?* Edinburgh: Cannogate Press.

Blom-Cooper, L. (1985) *A Child in Trust: Report of the Panel of Enquiry into the Circumstances Surrounding the Death of Jasmine Beckford*. London: Brent.

Booth, T. and Booth, W. (1994) *Parenting under Pressure, Mothers and Fathers with Learning Difficulties*. Buckingham: Open University Press.

Bowlby, J. (1969) *Attachment and Loss. Vol. 1: Attachment*. New York: Basic Books.

Bowlby, J. (1973) *Attachment and Loss. Vol. 2: Separation, Anxiety and Anger*. London: Hogarth.

Bridge Child Care Consultancy Service (1991) *Sukina: An Evaluation Report of the Circumstances leading to her Death*. London: Bridge.

British Association of Social Workers (BASW) (1988) *A Code of Ethics for Social Work*. Birmingham: BASW.

British Medical Association (BMA) (1983) *Handbook of Medical Ethics*. London: BMA.

Brook, E. and Davis, A. (eds) (1985) *Women, the Family and Social Work*. London: Tavistock.

Brown, H.C. (1991) Lesbians, the state and social work practice, in M. Langan and L. Day (eds) *Women, Oppression and Social Work: Issues in Anti Discriminatory Practice*. London: Routledge.

Brown, Justice (1991) Judgement on Rochdale child sexual abuse investigation, 1990. *Daily Telegraph*, 8 March: 3.

Bryan, A. (1991) Working with black single mothers: myths and reality, in M. Langan and L. Day (eds) *Women, Oppression and Social Work: Issues in Anti Discriminatory Practice*. London: Routledge.

Butler-Sloss, E. (1988) *Report of the Enquiry into Child Abuse in Cleveland, 1987*. London: HMSO.

Carlson, N.R. (1990) *Psychology. The Science of Behaviour* (3rd edn). Boston, London: Allyn and Bacon.

Carter, P., Everitt, A. and Hudson, A. (1992) Malestream training? in M. Langan and L. Day (eds) *Women, Oppression and Social Work: Issues in Anti Discriminatory Practice*. London: Routledge.

Carvalho, R. (1990) Psychodynamic therapy: the Jungian approach, in W. Dryden (ed.) *Individual Therapy*. Milton Keynes and Philadelphia: Open University Press.

Catania, A.C. (1992) *Learning* (3rd edn). Englewood Cliffs, NJ: Prentice Hall.

Channel 4 (1994a) *Dispatches*, 2 February

Channel 4 (1994b) *True Story*, 26 May.

Charles, N. (1993) *Gender Divisions and Social Change*. Hemel Hempstead and New York: Harvester Wheatsheaf, Barnes and Noble.

Clarke, K., Glendinning, C. and Craig, G. (1994) *Losing Support: Children and the Child Support Act*. London, Children's Society.

Clyde, Lord (1993) *Report of the Enquiry into the Removal of Children from Orkney in February 1991*. House of Commons, Session 1992/93, Paper 195. London: HMSO.

Collins English Dictionary (3rd edn) (1991) Harper Collins Publishers.

Connors, K.A., Heisner, L. and Trickett, P. (1992) CAPINDEX: Abstract descriptors. *Journal of Family Violence*, 4: 321–34.

Cooper, C. (1990) Psychodynamic therapy: the Kleinian approach, in W. Dryden (ed.) *Individual Therapy*. Milton Keynes and Philadelphia: Open University Press.

Cooper, D. (1993) *Child Abuse Revisited*. Buckingham: Open University Press.

Cooper, J.O., Heron, T.E. and Heward, W.I. (1987) *Applied Behavior Analysis*. Columbus, London: Merrill.

Coulshed, V. (1991) *Social Work Practice: An Introduction*. London: Macmillan.

Crampton, R. (1994) Leading the blind, *The Times Magazine*, 28 May.

Crittenden, P.M. (1990) Internal representation models of attachment relationships. *Journal of Infant Mental Health*, 11: 259–77.

Crittenden, P.M. and Ainsworth, M.D.S. (1989) Child maltreatment and attachment theory, in D. Cicchetti and V. Carlson (eds) *Child Maltreatment: Theory and Research on the Causes and Consequences of Child Abuse and Neglect*. New York: Cambridge University Press.

Currer, C. (1991) Understanding the mother's viewpoint: the case of Pathan women in Britain, in S. Wyke and J. Hewison (eds) *Child Health Matters*. Milton Keynes: Open University Press.

Daines, R., Lyon, K. and Parsloe, P. (1990) *Aiming for Partnership*. Essex: Barnardo's.

Dale, P., Davies, M., Morrison, T. and Waters, J. (1986) *Dangerous Families*. London: Tavistock.

Davies, J. (ed.), Berger, G. and Carlson, A. (1993) *The Family: Is it just another Lifestyle Choice?* London: The IEA Health and Welfare Unit.

Davies, M. (1991) Sociology and social work: a misunderstood relationship, in M. Davies (ed.) *The Sociology of Social Work*. London: Routledge.

Day, L. (1992) Women and oppression: race, class, and gender, in M. Langam and L. Day (eds) *Women, Oppression and Social Work: Issues in Anti Discriminatory Practice*. London: Routledge.

Deibert, A.N. and Harmon, A.J. (1978) *New Tools for Changing Behavior*. Illinois: Research Press.

Dennis, N. and Erdos, G. (1993) *Families Without Fatherhood*. London: The IEA Health and Welfare Unit.

Dennis, W. (1993) Untreue in den 90er Jahren: Die Frauen holen auf. *Psychologie Heute*, 10: 20–7.

Department of Health (DoH) (1988) *Protecting Children: A Guide for Social Workers undertaking a Comprehensive Assessment*. London: HMSO.

Department of Health (DoH) (1991a) *Child Abuse: A Study of Inquiry Reports 1980–1989*. London: HMSO.

Department of Health (DoH) (1991b) *Working Together*. London: HMSO.

Department of Health (DoH) (1993) *Adoption: The Future*. Cmnd. 2288. London: HMSO.

Department of Health and Social Security (DHSS) (1974) *Report of the Committee of Enquiry into the Care and Supervision Provided in Relation to Maria Colwell*. London: HMSO.

Department of Health and Social Security (DHSS) (1982) *Child Abuse: A Study of Enquiry Reports, 1973–81*. London: HMSO.

Dillenburger, K. and Keenan, M. (1993) Mummy don't leave me: The management of brief separation. *Practice*. British Association of Social Workers, 1: 66–9.

Dillenburger, K. and Keenan, M. (1994a) Smacking children: Dangers of misguided and outdated applications of psychological principles. *The Irish Psychologist*, 6: 56–8.

Dillenburger, K. and Keenan, M. (1994b) Bereavement: A behavioural process. *Irish Journal of Psychology*, 15: 324–39.

Dobrin, A. (1989) Ethical judgements of male and female social workers. *Social Work*, September: 451–5.

Dobson, R. (1994) The camera never lies. *Community Care*, 9–15 June: 26–7.

Dominelli, L. and McLeod, E. (1989) *Feminist Social Work*. Basingstoke: Macmillan.

Donnan, C. (1991) Domestic violence. *Domestic Violence and the Law*. Belfast: Conference held at the Law Society House.

Equal Opportunities Commission (for Northern Ireland) (1993) *Sexual Harassment at Work. Guidance on Prevention and Procedures for Dealing with the Problem*.

Erikson, E.H. (1963) *Childhood and Society*. New York: Norton.

Evason, E. (1980a) *Ends that Won't Meet*. London: Child Poverty Action Group.

Evason, E. (1980b) *Just Me and the Kids*. Belfast: Equal Opportunities Commission for NI.

Faludi, S. (1992) *Backlash: The Undeclared War Against Women*. London: Vintage.

Farmer, E. (1993) The impact of child protection interventions, in L. Waterhouse (ed.) *Child Abuse and Child Abusers*. London: Jessica Kingsley.

Ferguson, H. (1993) The manifest and latent implications of the report of the Kilkenny incest investigation. *Irish Social Worker*, 11(4): 4–7.

Figes, K. (1994) *Because of Her Sex: The Myth of Equality for Women in Britain*. London: Macmillan.

Finer, M. (1974) *Report of the Committee on One Parent Families*. Cmnd. 5629. London: HMSO.

Fox, Detective Inspector (1994) Independent detective work is not the best, letter in *Community Care*, 17 March.

Francis, J. (1992) At home in the grange. *Community Care*, 24 September.

French, M. (1993) *War Against Women*. New York: Summit Books.

Furniss, T. (1991) *The Multiprofessional Handbook of Child Sex Abuse. Integrated Management, Therapy and Legal Intervention*. London, New York: Routledge.

Gavron, H. (1968) *The Captive Wife. Conflicts of Housebound Mothers*. England, Australia: Pelican Books.

Gelfand, D.M. and Hartman D.P. (1986) *Child Behavior Analysis and Therapy* (2nd edn). Oxford: Pergamon Press.

Gewirtz, J.L. (1991) Social influence on child and parent via stimulation and operant-learning mechanisms, in M. Lewis and S. Feinman (eds) *Social Influences and Socialization in Infancy*. New York, London: Plenum Press.

Gewirtz, J.L. and Boyd, E.F. (1977) Experiments on mother–infant interaction underlying mutual attachment acquisition: The infant conditions the mother, in T. Alloway, P. Pliner and L. Krames (eds) *Attachment Behavior*. New York: Plenum.

Gewirtz, J.L. and Kurtines, W.M. (eds) (1991) *Intersections with Attachment*. Hillsdale, NJ: Lawrence Erlbaum.

Gewirtz, J.L. and Peláez-Nogueras, M. (1991) Proximal mechanisms underlying the acquisition of moral behavior patterns, in W.M. Kurtines and J.L. Gewirtz (eds) *Handbook of Moral Behavior and Development*. Hove, London: Lawrence Erlbaum.

Gewirtz, J.L. and Peláez-Nogueras, M. (1992) B.F. Skinner's legacy to human infant behavior and development. *American Psychologist*, 47: 1411–22.

Gillon, R. (1992) *Philosophical Medical Ethics*. West Sussex: Wiley.

Goddard, C. (1988) Point and Counterpoint: Child Statistical Abuse. *Australian Child And Family Welfare*. 12(4): 18–19.

Goddard, C. (1994) Still in the dark over the family raids. *The Age*, Melbourne, Australia, 6 May.

Goodacre, I. (1966) *Adoption Policy and Practice*. London: Allen and Unwin.

Gordon, T. (1990) *Feminist Mothers*. London: Macmillan.

Gragiano, A.M. (ed.) (1971) *Behavior Therapy With Children*. New York: Adline Atherton.

Granada Television (1993) *World in Action*, 4 October.

Grant, L. and Evans, A. (1994) *Principles of Behavior Analysis*. New York: Harper Collins.

Greenwich (1987) *Protection of Children in a Responsible Society: The Report of the Commission of Enquiry into the Circumstances Surrounding the Death of Kimberly Carlile*. London Borough of Greenwich, Greenwich Health Authority.

Grimwood, C. and Popplestone, R. (1993) *Women, Management and Care*. London: Macmillan.

Guerin, B. (1994) *Analysing Social Behavior. Behavior Analysis and the Social Sciences*. Reno: Context Press.

Hanmer, J. and Maynard, M. (eds) (1987) *Women, Violence and Social Control*. London: Macmillan.

Hanmer, J. and Statham, D. (1988) *Women and Social Work. Towards a Woman-Centred Practice*. London: Macmillan.

Hayes, L.J., Hayes, G.J., Moore, S.C. and Ghezzi, P.M. (eds) (1994) *Ethical Issues in Developmental Disabilities*. Reno: Context Press.

Hayes, M. (1992) *R v Devon County Council, Ex Parte L*, Bad practice, bad law and a breach of human rights. *Family Law*, June: 245–51.

Hayes, S.C., Hayes, L.J., Sato, A. and Ono, K. (eds) (1994) *Behavior Analysis of Language and Cognition*. Reno: Context Press.

Hayes, S.C. and Brownstein, A.J. (1986) Mentalism, behavior–behavior relations, and a behavior-analytic view of the purpose of science. *The Behavior Analyst*, 9: 175–90.

Hearn, J. (1990) Child abuse and men's violence. *Violence Against Children Study Group: Taking Child Abuse Seriously*. London: Unwin.

Hegarty, M. (1993) Women deserve more. *Irish Social Worker*, 11(4): 8–9.

Hendry, A. and Scourfield, F. (1994) Unanswered Questions. *Community Care*, 14 May.

Herbert, M. (1978) *Conduct Disorders of Childhood and Adolescence: A Behavioural Approach to Assessment and Treatment*. Chichester: John Wiley.

Herbert, M. (1986) *Psychology for Social Workers*. London: Macmillan.

Herbert, M. (1989) *Behavioural Treatment with Problem Children*. London: Academic Press.

Holland, J.G. (1978) Behaviorism: Part of the problem or part of the solution? *Journal of Applied Behavior Analysis*, 11: 27–38.

Holman, R. (1988) *Putting Families First*. London: Macmillan.

Hooper, C.-A. (1992) *Mothers Surviving Child Sexual Abuse*. London: Routledge.

Horley, S. (1990) A Shame and a Disgrace. *Social Work Today*, 41: 16–17.

Houghton, W. (1972) *Report of the Departmental Committee on the Adoption of Children*. Cmnd. 5107. London: HMSO.

Howe, A.C., Herzberger, S. and Tennen, H. (1988) The influence of personal history of abuse and gender on clinicians' judgements of child abuse. *Journal of Family Violence*, 3(2): 105–19.

Howe, D. (1987) *An Introduction to Social Work Theory*. Aldershot: Wildwood House.

Howe, D., Sawbridge, P. and Hinings, D. (1992) *Half a Million Women: Mothers Who Lose Their Children By Adoption*. London: Penguin.

Howitt, D. (1992) *Child Abuse Errors: When Good Intentions Go Wrong*. Hemel Hempstead: Harvester Wheatsheaf.

Hudson, A. (1993) The child sexual abuse 'industry' and gender relations in social work, in M. Lagan and L. Day (eds) *Women, Oppression and Social Work: Issues in Anti Discriminatory Practice*. London, New York: Routledge.

Hudson, A., Ayonsi, L., Oadley, C. and Patocchi, M. (1994) Practising feminist approaches, in C. Hanvey and T. Philpot (eds) *Practising Social Work*. London: Routledge.

Hudson, B.L. and McDonald, G.M. (1991) *Behavioural Social Work. An Introduction*. Basingstoke: Macmillan.

Jackson, S. (1993) Family fortunes. *Community Care*, 9 December.

Jaffe, P.G., Wolfe, D.A. and Wilson, S.K. (1990) *Children of Battered Women*. New York: Sage.

Janchill, Sr. M.P. (1969) Systems in casework theory and practice. *Social Casework*, 50(2), republished in W. Klenk and R.M. Ryan (eds) (1970) *The Practice of Social Work*. USA: Wadworth.

Jason, L.A. (1984) Developing undergraduates' skills in behavioral interventions. *Journal of Community Psychology*, 12: 130–9.

Johnston, J.M. and Sherman, R.A. (1993) Applying the least restrictive alternative principle to treatment decisions: A legal and behavioral analysis. *The Behavior Analyst*, 16: 103–15.

Kahan, B. (1979) *Growing Up in Care*. Oxford, Basil Blackwell.

Keenan, M. (1991) W-ing. Teaching exercises for radical behaviourists. Unpublished paper. University of Ulster at Coleraine.

Keenan, M. (1993) For evil to persist all it takes is for good men to do nothing: Dealing with misrepresentations of a caring profession. *The Irish Psychologist*, 11: 34.

Kelly, G. (1989) Patterns of care: the first twelve months. *Personal Social Services in Northern Ireland*, 37, January.

Kempe, R.S. and Kempe, C.H. (1978) *Child Abuse*. London: Fontana Open Books.

King, M. and Trowell, J. (1992) *Children's Welfare and the Law: the Limits of Legal Intervention*. London: Sage.

Kirwan, M. (1994) Gender and social work: will Dip.S.W. make a difference? *British Journal of Social Work*, 24: 137–55.

Lambert, L., Buist, M. and Triseliotis, J. (1989) *Freeing Children for Adoption: Summary of the Main Findings*. ssn. 0950–2250, Scottish Office: HMSO.

Lambeth (1987) *Whose Child? The Report of the Public Enquiry into the Death of Tyra Henry*. London Borough of Lambeth.

Langan, M. (1991a) Introduction: women and social work in the 1990s, in M. Langan and L. Day (eds) *Women, Oppression and Social Work: Issues in Anti Discriminatory Practice*. London, New York: Routledge.

Langan, M. (1991b) Who cares? Women in the mixed economy of care, in M. Langan and L. Day (eds) *Women, Oppression and Social Work: Issues in Anti Discriminatory Practice*. London, New York: Routledge.

Langan, M. and Day, L. (eds) (1992) *Women, Oppression and Social Work: Issues in Anti Discriminatory Practice*. London, New York: Routledge.

LaVigna, G.W. and Donnellan, A.M. (1986) *Alternatives to Punishment: Solving Behavior Problems with Non-Aversive Strategies*. New York: Irvington.

Law Commission (1992) *Criminal Law, Rape within Marriage*. London: HMSO, 13 January.

Lawrence, M. (1992) Women's psychology and feminist social work practice, in M. Langan and L. Day (eds) *Women, Oppression and Social Work: Issues in Anti Discriminatory Practice*. London, New York: Routledge.

Leeds City Council (1990) *Press Release Bogus Social Workers*. Leeds.

Levy, A. and Kahan, B. (1991) *The Pindown Experience and the Protection of Children: A Report of the Staffordshire Child Care Inquiry*. Staffordshire: Staffordshire County Council.

Little, W., Fowler, H.W. and Coulson J. (1983) *The Shorter Oxford English Dictionary*, London: Guild.

Lloyd, K.E. (1994a) Do as I say, not as I do. *The Behavior Analyst*, 17: 131–9.

Lloyd, K.E. (1994b) Addenda. *The Behavior Analyst*, 17: 141–4.

Lorber, J. and Farrell, S.A. (eds) (1991) *The Social Construction of Gender*. Beverly Hills: Sage.

Lowe, N. (1993) *Report of the Research in the Use and Practice of Freeing For Adoption Provisions*. London: HMSO.

Lundin, R.W. (1969) *Personality: An experimental approach*. New York: Macmillan.

Lupton, C. (1991) Feminism, managerialism and performance measurement, in M. Langan and L. Day (eds) *Women, Oppression and Social Work: Issues in Anti Discriminatory Practice*. London, New York: Routledge.

McAuley, P. (1981) Teaching behaviour therapy skills to social work students. *British Journal of Social Work*, 11: 203–15.

McBeath, G. and Webb, S. (1990–1) Child protection language and professional ideology in social work. *Social Work and Social Sciences Review*, 2(2): 122–45.

McGoldrick, M. (1989) Women and the family life cycle, in B. Carter and M.

McGoldrick (eds) *The Changing Family Life Cycle. A Framework for Family Therapy*. London, Boston: Allyn and Bacon.

McLaughlin, I.G., Leonard, K.E. and Senack, M. (1992) Prevalence and distribution of premarital aggression among couples applying for a marriage license. *Journal of Family Violence*, 4: 309–19.

McLeod, L. and Dominelli, L. (1982) The personal and the apolitical: feminism and moving beyond the integrated methods approach, in R. Baily and P. Lees (eds) *Theory and Practice in Social Work*. Oxford: Basil Blackwell.

McMinn, K. (1991) Effective intervention in domestic violence. *Domestic Violence and the Law*. Belfast: Conference held at the Law Society House.

McNay, M. (1991) Social work and power relations: towards a framework for integrated practice, in M. Langan and L. Day (eds) *Women, Oppression and Social Work: Issues in Anti Discriminatory Practice*. London, New York: Routledge.

McShane, L. and Pinkerton, J. (1986) The family in Northern Ireland. *Studies*, 75: 167–76.

McWilliams, M. and McKiernan, J. (1993) *Bringing It Out in the Open: Domestic Violence in Northern Ireland*. London: HMSO.

Malcolm, S. and O'Hagan, K.P. (1994) *Parental/Carer Perceptions and Professional Perspectives of the Child Protection Process*. Second National Congress of BASPCAN, Bristol, 5–8 July.

Malott, R.W. and Whaley, D.L. (1983) *Psychology*. Holmes Beach, Fla.: Learning Publications.

Malott, R.W., Whaley, D.L. and Malott, M.E. (1993) *Elementary Principles of Behavior*. Englewood Cliffs, NJ: Prentice Hall.

Martin, G. and Pear, J. (1992) *Behaviour Modification. What It Is and How to Do It*. New York: Simon and Schuster.

Mash, E.J., Hammerlynck, L.A. and Handy, L.C. (eds) (1976) *Behaviour Modification and Families*. New York: Brunner/Mazel.

Meadows, R. (1985) Management of Munchausen syndrome by proxy. *Archives of Disease in Childhood*, 60: 385–93.

Meadows, R. (1993a) False allegations of abuse and Munchausen syndrome by proxy. *Archives of Disease in Childhood*, 68: 444–7.

Meadows, R. (1993b) Non-accidental salt poisoning. *Archives of Disease and Medicine*, 68: 448–52.

Michael, J.L. (1993) *Concepts and Principles of Behavior Analysis*. Kalamazoo: Society for the Advancement of Behavior Analysis.

Miles, A. (1991) *Women, Health and Medicine*. Buckingham: Open University Press.

Millenson, J.R. and Leslie, J.C. (1979) *Principles of Behavioural Analysis* (2nd edn). New York: Macmillan.

Miller, J.B. (1976) *Towards a New Psychology of Women*. Harmondsworth: Penguin.

Millham, S., Bullock, R., Hosie, K. and Haak, M. (1986) *Lost in Care*. London: Gower.

Milner, J. (1993) A disappearing act: The differing career paths of fathers and mothers in child protection investigations. *Critical Social Policy*, 38: 48–63.

Minuchin, S. (1974) *Families and Family Therapy*. London: Tavistock.

Minuchin, S. and Fishman, H.C. (1981) *Family Therapy Techniques*. Cambridge, MA: Harvard University Press.

Moore, J. (1988) The question the Carlile report failed to answer. *Community Care*, 14 January.

Morley, C. (1992) Experts differ over diagnostic criteria for Munchausen syndrome by proxy. Letter in *British Journal of Hospital Medicine*, 48: 3–4.

Morris, E.K., Hursh, D.E., Winston, A.S., Gelfand, D.M., Hartmann, D.P., Reese, H.W. and Baer, D.M. (1982) Behavior analysis and developmental psychology. *Human Development*, 25: 340–64.

Myers, D.L. (1993) Participation by women in behavior analysis. *The Behavior Analyst*, 16: 75–86.

National Children's Bureau (NCB) (1993) *Investigation into Inter-Agency Practice Following the Cleveland Area Child Protection Committee's Report Concerning the Death of Toni Dales*. London: NCB.

National Institute for Social Work (1994) *Consultation on the DipSW Review of Competences for Professionally Qualified Social Workers*. Developed on behalf of Central Council for Education and Training in Social Work and the Care Sector Consortium, 6 July.

Neef, N.A. (ed.) (1994) Special issue on functional analysis approaches to behavioral assessment and treatment. *Journal of Applied Behavioral Analysis*, 27: 196–418.

Newman, T. (1993) Keeping in step. *Community Care*, 28 October.

Norris, D. (1991) *Violence Against Social Workers: The Implication for Practice*. London: Jessica Kingsley.

Nye, R.D. (1992) *The Legacy of B. F. Skinner. Concepts and Perspectives, Controversies and Misunderstandings*. California: Brooks/Cole.

Oakley, A. (1982) *Subject Women. A Powerful Analysis of Women's Experience in Society Today*. London: Fontana Paperbacks.

Observer, The (1991) Killed by her father, doomed by officialdom, 24 November.

Observer, The (1993) Fiction and the facts, 11 July.

Offences against the Person's Act (1861) in Law Commission (1992) *Criminal Law, Rape within Marriage*. London: HMSO, 13 January.

O'Hagan, K.P. (1984) Family crisis intervention in social services. *Journal of Family Therapy*, 6: 149–81.

O'Hagan, K.P. (1986) There isn't an effective crisis training program. *Social Work Today*, 29 September.

O'Hagan, K.P. (1989) *Working with Child Sexual Abuse*. Milton Keynes: Open University Press.

O'Hagan, K.P. (1990) When experts build a rotten foundation. *Social Work Today*, 30 November.

O'Hagan, K.P. (1991) Crisis intervention in social work, in J. Lishman (ed.) *Handbook of Theory and Practice for Social Work*. London: Jessica Kingsley.

O'Hagan, K.P. (1993) *Emotional and Psychological Abuse of Children*. Buckingham: Open University Press.

O'Hagan, K.P. (1994a) Crisis intervention: Changing perspectives, in C. Hanvey and T. Philpot (eds) *Practising Social Work*. London: Routledge.

O'Hagan K.P. (1994b) *Parental participation in emergency child protection work and case conferences*. Paper presented to 10th International Congress on Child Abuse and Neglect, Kuala Lumpur, Malaysia.

Page, R. and Clarke, G. (eds) (1977) *Who Cares? Young People in Care Speak Out*. London: NCB.

PAIN (Parents Against Injustice) (1987) *PAIN's Statement to the Cleveland Enquiry*, December. Essex: PAIN.

PAIN (1990a) Details on concerns about the failure to carry out good practice in Rochdale (and elsewhere) as recommended by *Working Together* and the *Code of Practice-Access to Children in Care*. Essex: PAIN.

PAIN (1990b) *Report and Recommendations on Voluntary and Compulsory Ousting*. Essex: PAIN.

Parton, C. (1990) Women, gender oppression and child abuse, in the *Violence Against Children Study Group: Taking Child Abuse Seriously*. London: Unwin.

Pearce, N. (1984) *Adoption Practice and Procedure*. London: Fourmat.

Phares, V. (1992) Where's Poppa? The relative lack of attention to the role of fathers in child and adolescent psychopathology. *American Psychologist*, 5: 656–64.

Phillips, R. (1993) Stepping into a family. *Community Care*, 24 June.

Piaget, J. (1954) *The Construction of Reality in the Child*. New York: Basic Books.

Pick, P. (1981) *Children at Tree Tops: An example of Creative Residential Care*. London: Residential Care Association.

Pilgrim, D. and Rogers, A. (1993) *A Sociology of Mental Illness*. Buckingham: Open University Press.

Pinkerton, J. (1994) Advocacy means? *Child Care Northern Ireland*, 5: 3.

Pinkston, E.M., Levitt, J.L., Green, G.R., Linsk, N.L. and Rzepnicki, T.L. (1982) *Effective Social Work Practice*. London, Washington: Jossey-Bass.

Poling, A., Schlinger, H., Starin, S. and Blakely, E. (1990) *Psychology: A Behavioral Overview*. New York: Plenum Press.

Popay, J. (1992) My health is all right, but I'm just tired all the time, in H. Roberts (ed) *Women's Health Matters*. London: Routledge.

Pryor, K. (1984) *Don't Shoot the Dog. The New Art of Teaching and Training*. New York, London: Bantam.

Quinn, O. (1991) The legal response to domestic violence. *Domestic Violence and the Law*. Belfast: Conference held at the Law Society House.

Rachlin, H. (1991) *Introduction to Modern Behaviorism*. New York: W.H. Freeman.

Ramazanoglu, C. (1987) Sex and violence in academic life or you can keep a good woman down, in J. Hanmer and M. Maynard (eds) *Women, Violence and Social Control*. London: Macmillan.

Reder, P., Duncan, S. and Gray, M. (1993) *Beyond Blame; Child Abuse Tragedies Revisited*. London: Routledge.

Reese, E.P., with Howard, J. and Reese, T.W. (1978) *Human Operant Behavior. Analysis and Application* (2nd edn) Iowa: Wm. C. Brown.

Reich, D. (1988) *Working With Mothers who Lost a Child Through Adoption*. London: Post Adoption Centre.

Reynolds, S. (ed.) (1986) *Women, State and Revolution. Essays on Power and Gender in Europe since 1789*. Brighton: Wheatsheaf.

Richardson, S. and Bacon, H. (1991) *Child Sexual Abuse, Whose Problem? Reflections From Cleveland*. Birmingham: Venture.

Rickford, F. (1992) Courting danger. *Social Work Today*, 8 October.

Rickford, F. (1993) Hit and myth. *Community Care*, 9 December.

Ridd, R. and Callaway, H. (eds) (1986) *Caught Up in Conflict. Women's Response to Political Strife*. London: Macmillan.

Riggs, D.S., Kilpatrick, D.G. and Resnick, H.S. (1992) Long-term psychological distress associated with marital rape and aggravated assault: A comparison to other crime victims. *Journal of Family Violence*, 4: 283–96.

Robertson, I. (1993) Whose law is it anyway? *Community Care*, 7 October.

Robinson, J.J. (1991) Domestic violence intervention – The Canadian experience. *Domestic Violence and the Law*. Belfast: Conference held at the Law Society House.

Rosales, J. and Baer, D.M. (in press) A behavior-analytic view of development, in E. Ribes and S.W. Bijou (eds) *Recent Approaches to Behavioral Development*. Jal, México: Guadalajara.

Ross, M. and Glisson, C. (1991) Bias in social work intervention with battered women. *Journal of Social Services Research*, 14(3/4): 79–105.

Rowe, J. and Lambert, L. (1973) *Children Who Wait*. London: Association of British Adoption Agencies.

Rowett, C. (1986) *Violence in Social Work*. Cambridge: University of Cambridge Institute of Criminology.

Russel, R., Gill, P., Coyne, A. and Woody, J. (1993) Dysfunction in the family of origin of MSW and other graduate students. *Journal of Social Work Education*, 29(1): 121–9.

Sayers, J. (1991) Blinded by family feeling? Child protection, feminism, and counter-transference, in P.Carter, T. Jeffs and M. Smith (eds) *Social Work and Social Welfare Yearbook 3*. Buckingham: Open University Press.

Schlinger, H.D. (1992) Theory in behavior analysis. An application to child development. *American Psychologist*, 11: 1396–410.

Schorr, L.B. with Schorr, D. (1989) *Within our Reach. Breaking the Cycle of Disadvantage*. London, New York: Anchor Books, Doubleday.

Scott, J. and Tilly, L. (1982) Women's work and the family in nineteenth-century Europe, in E. Whitelegg, M. Arnot, E. Bartels, V. Beechey, L. Birke, S. Himmelweit, D. Leonard, S. Ruehl and M. A. Speakman (eds) *The Changing Experience of Women*. Oxford: Martin Robertson in association with The Open University Press.

Sexual Offences Act (1956) In Law Commission (1992) *Criminal Law, Rape within Marriage*. London: HMSO, 13 January.

Sexual Offences (Amendment) Act (1976) In Law Commission (1992) *Criminal Law, Rape within Marriage*. London: HMSO, 13 January.

Seward, G.H. and Williamson, R.C. (1970) *Sex Roles in Changing Society*. New York: Random House.

Shawyer, J. (1979) *Death by Adoption*. Auckland: Cicado Press.

Sidman, M. (1989) *Coercion and its Fallout*. Boston: Author's Cooperative.

Skinner, B.F. (1953) *Science and Human Behavior*. New York: Macmillan.

Skinner, B.F. (1989) *Recent Issues in the Analysis of Behavior*. Columbus, Ohio: Merrill.

Smith, D. (1990) Psychodynamic therapy: the Freudian approach, in W. Dryden (ed.) *Individual Therapy*. Milton Keynes and Philadelphia: Open University Press.

Social Services Inspectorate (SSI) (1993) *Corporate Parents: Inspection of Residential Child Care Services in 11 Local Authorities*. London: Department of Health.

Sommerfeld, D.P. and Hughes, J.R. (1987) Do health professionals agree on the parenting potential of pregnant women? *Social Sciences Medicine*, 24(3): 285–8.

Sone, K. (1993) Mother's help. *Community Care,*15 April.

Staats, A. (1994) Psychological behaviorism and behaviorizing psychology. *The Behavior Analyst,* 17: 93–114.

Statham, D. (1987) Women, the new right, and social work. *Journal of Social Work Practice,* 2(4): 129–49.

Stephenson, T. (1994) The hand that rocks the cradle. *Community Care,* 10 March.

Stockard, J. and Johnson, M.M. (1980) *Sex roles. Sex Inequality and Sex Role Development.* Englewood Cliffs, NJ: Prentice Hall.

Strachney, J. (ed.) (1963) *The Standard Edition of the Complete Works of S. Freud.* London: Hogarth Press.

Sulzer-Azaroff, B. and Mayer, G.R. (1991) *Behavior Analysis for Lasting Change.* New York, London: Holt, Rinehart and Winston.

Sulzer-Azaroff, B. and Reese, E. (1982) *Applying Behavior Analysis: A Program for Developing Professional Competence.* New York: Holt, Rinehart and Winston.

Terry, J. (1976) *A Guide to the Children Act, 1975.* London: Sweet and Maxwell.

Thoburn, J. (1992) *Participation in Practice Involving Parents in Child Protection.* Norwich: University of East Anglia.

Thoburn, J. (1993) The adoption prism. *Community Care,* 24 June.

Thomas, T. (1994) Court video surveillance. *New Law Journal,* 15 July: 966–7.

Thorpe, D. (1994) Facing reality. *Community Care,* 31 August: 32–3.

Triseliotis, J. (1989) Foster care outcomes: A review of key research findings. *Adoption and Fostering,* 1: 3.

Triseliotis, J. (1993) Keeping in touch. *Community Care,* 24 June.

Triseliotis, J. and Hall, E. (1971) Giving consent to adoption. *Social Work Today,* 2(17): 21–4.

United Kingdom Central Council for Nursing, Midwifery and Health Visiting (1992) *Code of Professional Conduct.* London: UKCC.

Urwin, C. (1985) Constructing motherhood: The persuasion of normal development, in C. Steedman, C. Urwin and V. Walkerdine (eds) *Language, Gender and Childhood.* London: Routledge and Kegan Paul.

Van Houten, R., Axelrod, S., Bailey, J.S., Favell, J.E., Foxx, R.M., Iwata, B.A. and Lovaas, O.I. (1988) *The Right to Effective Treatment.* Kalamazoo: Association for Behavior Analysis.

Walrond-Skinner, S. (1976) *Family Therapy: The Treatment of Natural Systems.* London: Routledge and Kegan Paul.

Walton, R.G. (1975) *Women in Social Work.* London, Boston: Routledge and Kegan Paul.

Wertheimer, A. (1987) Sterilization: for better or for worse. *Childright,* 38: 17–19.

Westminster College (1992) *Child Abuse: The Families' Perspective.* Oxford: Westminster College.

Wheeler, H. (ed.) (1973) *Beyond the Punitive Society. Operant Conditioning: Social and political aspects.* San Francisco: W. H. Freeman.

Whitelegg, E., Arnot, M., Bartels, E., Beechey, V., Birke, L., Himmelweit, S., Leonard, D., Ruehl, S. and Speakman, M.A. (eds) (1982) *The Changing Experience of Women.* Oxford: Martin Robertson in association with The Open University Press.

Williams, F. (1991) Women with learning difficulties are women too, in M. Langan and L. Day (eds) *Women, Oppression and Social Work: Issues in Anti Discriminatory Practice*. London, New York: Routledge.

Winkler, R. and Van Kepple, M. (1984) *Relinquishing Mothers in Adoption: Their Long-Term Adjustment*. Melbourne: Institute of Family Studies.

Wise, S. and Stanley, L. (1990) Sexual harassment, sexual conduct and gender in social work. *Social Work and Social Welfare Yearbook*. Buckingham: Open University Press.

Zimbardo, P.G. (1988) *Psychology and Life* (12th edn). Boston, London: Scott Foresman.

Zito, J. (1994) MIND should wake up to the facts of violence. *Community Care* (Letter to Editor), 14–20 July.

Index